BACH
FLOWER THERAPY

The latest and most comprehensive book on the Bach
Flower Remedies which, as well as describing the 38
remedies, goes into the spiritual and psychological
applications of the therapy so that both patients and
practitioners can gain deeper insight into the underlying
concepts.

BACH
FLOWER
THERAPY
Theory and Practice

by

Mechthild Scheffer

*(Translated from the German
by A.R. Meuss F.I.L., M.T.G.)*

THORSONS PUBLISHING GROUP

First published in Germany as *Die Bach Blütentherapie* 1981 revised 1984

© Heinrich Hugendubel Verlag, München, West Germany 1981

First published in English 1986

© THORSONS PUBLISHING GROUP LIMITED 1986

British Library Cataloguing in Publication Data

Scheffer, Mechthild
The Bach flower therapy: theory and practice.
1. Materia medica, vegetable
I. Title   II. Die Bach Blütentherapie, English
615'.32   RS164

ISBN 0-7225-1121-3

*Published by Thorsons Publishers Limited,
Wellingborough, Northamptonshire, NN8 2RQ, England*

Printed in Great Britain by Woolnough Bookbinding,
Irthlingborough, Northamptonshire

5   7   9   10   8   6   4

CONTENTS

INTRODUCTION

This book was originally written at the request and suggestion of my patients and colleagues in German speaking countries who wished to know more about Bach Flower Therapy. It is based on fourteen years of extensive experience into the Bach Flower Remedies as well as an evaluation of the available literature on the subject.

It was the wish of the man who discovered the method, the Harley Street physician Dr Edward Bach, that this form of healing by means of wild flowers should be accessible not only to the medical profession but also to lay people with no medical training.

The thirty-eight flowers are described in depth, so that patients taking one of them may also gain further understanding of the underlying concept in each case, to strengthen the self-healing process.

It is important to note, for all readers who are not trained in medicine, that the Bach Flower Remedies may be employed to prevent psychological and physical illness and in support of prescribed treatment, but cannot be used to replace treatment by a qualified medical practitioner.

The author would like to express her gratitude to all the people, at home and abroad, who have contributed to the writing of this book, and particularly also for the co-operation and support received from the Bach Centre in England, the only place where the Bach Flower Remedies are still prepared from wild flowers, using the same locations and the original methods that Dr Edward Bach had found over fifty years ago.

Mechthild Scheffer
Hamburg, 1986

Chapter 1

THE BACH FLOWER REMEDIES — A HOLISTIC APPROACH TO TREATMENT

'Disease is solely and purely corrective; it is neither vindictive nor cruel, but it is the means adopted by our own souls to point out to us our faults, to prevent our making greater errors, to hinder us from doing more harm, and to bring us back to the path of Truth and Light from which we should never have strayed.'

The timeless reality of this statement, made by the English physician Dr Edward Bach more than fifty years ago, is being increasingly realized in this era of the 'New Age', of 'humanized', 'psychosomatic' and 'holistic' medicine, and internationally interest in the Bach Flower Remedies has been markedly renewed in recent years, as Dr Bach once predicted.

The holistic approach to health, disease and healing is based on the concept of the perfect Unity of all things, and the utter Uniqueness of every system contained within it. Each of us is on a unique and unrepeatable journey through life, and our state of health at any time serves as an indicator of the point we have reached on this journey.

Every symptom, be it of body, mind or spirit, gives us a particular message, and we need to perceive and acknowledge these messages, and make use of them for our journey. Every true healing process is an affirmation of our wholeness, indeed our holiness. The Bach Flower Remedies' system may from this point of view be described as 'healing by restoring harmony in awareness'. At the switch-points of our personality, where vital energies are channelled the wrong way or blocked, the remedies re-establish contact and harmony with our wholeness, the true source of our energy.

'Heal Thyself' is at the very heart of Edward Bach's philosophy, for in the final instance it is we ourselves, the 'universal principle of healing' or the 'divine healing power' within us, that permit and enable healing. It was Dr Bach's vision that his Flower Remedies would be used, not only by physicians and lay practitioners, but also in every family.

In this way, the Bach Flowers would not only be used by professionals in the treatment of psychosomatic disorders, but also and increasingly by people who are consciously working on their mental and spiritual growth and development.

The Bach Flower Remedies rank among the 'subtle' methods of healing, similar to the classical homoeopathy of Samuel Hahnemann, anthroposophical medicine, and spagyric or herbal medicine. They do not act by the roundabout route via the physical body, but at more subtle levels directly influencing the energy system that is man.

Before he developed his Flower Remedies, Edward Bach M.B., B.S., D.P.H., was a highly successful bacteriologist and homoeopathic physician*. He felt a spiritual link among others with Hippocrates, Paracelsus and Samuel Hahnemann, sharing their view that 'There are no diseases, but only sick people'. Yet it would be taking too narrow a view of him and his work if one were to call him the 'present-day Hahnemann', as contemporary colleagues have done.

It was in 1930 that Dr Bach, then aged 43, gave up his lucrative Harley Street practice, to devote the last six years of his life to the search for a simpler, more natural method of treatment that did not 'require anything to be destroyed or altered'.† Here was a quest that in many respects went beyond Hahnemann's outlook and aims.

There are three respects in which the Bach Flower Remedies are new and different from the subtle methods of treatment so far developed in the West:
1.   Edward Bach's concept of health and disease, i.e. the spiritual approach he uses, has its roots in a universal reference system that goes beyond the limits of the individual person.‡ This led him to a new form of

*The seven Bach nosodes he introduced have become a firmly established part of the international homoeopathic materia medica.

†Details of the person and life of Edward Bach may be found in the biography written by Nora Weeks, *The Medical Discoveries of Edward Bach, Physician*. (C.W. Daniel, 1940).

‡Set out in detail in no more than 52 pages in his main work, *Heal Thyself*. (C.W. Daniel, 1931).

diagnosis, no longer based on physical symptoms, but exclusively on states of disharmony in the soul, or negative feelings, similar to, but more comprehensive than, the homoeopathic 'mentals'.

2. New, and different in the present age, are also the simple, natural methods Bach used to release the healing energies of the flowers from their material state, and transfer them to the vehicle. As a result his Flower Remedies act directly, i.e. not according to the Law of Similars, harmonizing and healing, and there can be no overdosage, no side-effects, and no incompatibility with other methods of treatment.

3. This mode of action, 'harmless' in the best sense of the word, makes the blessings of Bach's Remedies accessible to a far greater number of people, to use in healing and self-healing, than has so far been possible with subtle healing methods. To use the Bach Remedies successfully calls for no training in medicine or psychology, but for perceptiveness, the ability to think and to appreciate, and above all a natural sensitivity and feeling for the other person.

Chapter 2

HOW DO THE REMEDIES WORK? — A POSSIBLE INTERPRETATION

To date, no explanation exists of the mode of action that would fully satisfy current scientific criteria. Hypotheses based on molecular chemistry, cybernetics and atomic physics have been put forward for other subtle healing methods. It is possible that these would also apply to the Bach Remedies. Considering the extremely rapid expansion of knowledge in these fields, it can only be a matter of time until the energy changes produced by these subtle methods can also be measured and demonstrated by scientific methods.

Edward Bach wrote down everything he considered important in relation to his method of treatment in just a few words in his two works *Heal Thyself* and *The Twelve Healers and Other Remedies* (both published by C.W. Daniel, Saffron Walden, Essex). Those familiar with his spiritual world will to this day need no more than these two booklets. And everybody who takes up the Bach Flower Remedies, whether therapist or patient ought to have his or her own copy of *Heal Thyself*, to read and reread.

It has been found, however, that today not everyone can grasp and accept the simplicity and greatness of Edward Bach's thoughts, written fifty years ago. Therefore his thoughts and the mode of action of the Flower Remedies are here presented and explained in the light of today's knowledge and perception.

This is supplemented with an interpretation of the action from a psycho-dynamic point of view, an approach often used by practitioners who consider the psychological aspects. Finally, for those who are interested, further insights gained in the practice of an esoteric healer are also presented.

A. EDWARD BACH'S INTERPRETATION
In 1934, Bach wrote the following concerning the way his Flower Remedies work:

> The action of these remedies is to raise our vibrations and open up our channels for the reception of the Spiritual Self; to flood our natures with the particular virtue we need, and wash out from us the fault that is causing the harm. They are able, like beautiful music or any glorious uplifting thing which gives us inspiration, to raise our very natures, and bring us nearer to our souls and by that very act to bring us peace and relieve our sufferings. They cure, not by attacking the disease, but by flooding our bodies with the beautiful vibrations of our Higher Nature, in the presence of which, disease melts away as snow in the sunshine.
>
> There is no true healing unless there is a change in outlook, peace of mind, and inner happiness.

To many people this may at first sound improbable, but it becomes perfectly clear if the premise on which Bach based his line of thought — similar to Hippocrates, Hahnemann and Paracelsus, great men of like spirit — is understood and accepted.

1. Creation and Destiny
Human life, man on this planet, is but part of a greater concept of creation. We live within a wider frame of reference, a more comprehensive unity, more or less like a cell within a human body. Every person is two things: a unique individual, and a vital and essential part of the greater unity, the greater whole.

Within creation, there is Unity in all things, and each of us is related to everything else by a common, higher, more powerful form of energy that has been given many names, for instance 'creative force', 'universal Life principle', 'cosmic principle', 'love' (in the sense of a higher form of reason), or simply 'God'.

Like everything else in our universe, from frost-patterns on our windows to the generation and death of whole planetary systems, the development of every individual human being follows a programmed course of action and reaction, an inherent law. Every human being has a matrix with specific energy potentials, has a mission, a task, a destiny, *karma*, or whatever we may call it.

Being part of the great plan of creation, every human being has an immortal Soul — his real Self — and a mortal Personality — that which he represents here on earth. There is a Higher Self which is closely bound up with his Soul and may be said to function as the mediator between Soul and Personality.

The Soul is aware of the particular mission a person has, and endeavours to bring this mission to expression, with the aid of the Higher Self and through the flesh and blood Personality, and make it a concrete reality. To begin with the Personality is not aware of this mission. The potentials our Soul wishes to bring to realization through the Personality are not concrete. They are in fact higher, ideal qualities that Edward Bach referred to as 'the virtues of our Higher Self'. They include gentleness, firmness, courage, constancy, wisdom, joyfulness, purposefulness. Poets of all ages have praised these as noble qualities of character. They could also be called the ideal archetypal soul qualities of mankind, the realization of which will lead to true happiness within the context of a greater Whole.

If these are not brought to realization, the opposite feeling, unhappiness, will sooner or later develop. The potential virtues which we have failed to realize now show themselves from their negative side, as 'defects' such as pride, cruelty, hatred, self-love, ignorance, greed. These defects, as not only Edward Bach tells us, are the true causes of disease. Every person has the unconscious desire to live in harmony, for nature, considered as a huge energy field, is always endeavouring to produce the most effective energy state.

2. Health and Disease

Health. If the personality could and would act wholly in harmony with its soul, which itself is part of the greater whole, man would be living in perfect harmony. The universal divine creative energy would be able to express itself through the Soul and the Higher Self in the Personality, and we would be strong, fit and happy people, our energies in harmony with the great cosmic energy field of which we are a part.

Disease. Wherever the Personality is not connected to the great cosmic energy field by its Soul, not swinging in harmony with it, there is disruption, congestion, friction, distortion, disharmony, loss of energy. These conditions are first present in subtle, non-material form, but then progress to the material level, manifesting first in the form of negative moods, and later in physical illness. The function of physical illness is that of a final corrective. To put it simply, it is a red warning light, very clearly indicating that something has to be done immediately, for otherwise total failure will follow sooner or later.

Edward Bach said that two basic errors are the real cause of disease:

The first error: The Personality is not acting in accord with its Soul, but persists in the illusion of being separate from it.

At the absolute extreme, the Personality is no longer in a position even to recognize the existence of the Soul and of a Higher Self, materialistically accepting only what 'can be seen and touched'. In the long run, it thus cuts its own umbilical cord, withers and destroys itself.

More often, however, the Personality merely misunderstands the Soul's intentions in certain respects, and then acts according to its limited understanding of the situation.

In all the separate areas where the Personality has turned away from the great cosmic energy flow, or from Love, as Edward Bach put it, virtues, i.e. positive character traits, are distorted and become destructive, leading to negative soul states and moods.*

The second error: The Personality sins against the 'Principle of Unity'. By acting against the intentions of its Higher Self and Soul, the Personality is automatically also acting against the interests of the Greater Unity, its Soul being linked to it in terms of energy.

Above all, however, the Personality is sinning against the Principle of Unity if it attempts to force its own will on another being, against the will of the latter. This not only impedes the development of the other, but also, all things being related, upsets the whole cosmic energy field, i.e. the development of mankind as a whole.

Any illness is preceded by a negative state of soul, due to one of the great archetypal human soul qualities or virtues

---

*'Righteousness without love makes us hard. Faith without love makes us fanatical. Power without love makes us brutal. Duty without love makes us peevish. Orderliness without love makes us petty'. This anonymous quotation puts it perfectly.

being misused. Here is an example:

The negative state of soul might be inconsiderate, egotistical attitudes, arising from greed as a wrongly used virtue. Greed is the negative side of the soul quality of love for one's neighbour and tolerance.

In *Heal Thyself*, Edward Bach wrote: 'Greed leads to a desire for power. It is a denial of the freedom and individuality of every soul. Instead of recognizing that every one of us is here to develop freely upon his own lines according to the dictates of the soul alone, to increase his individuality, and to work free and unhampered, the personality with greed desires to dictate, mould and command, usurping the power of the Creator.

'... Each of such defects, if persisted in against the voice of the Higher Self, will produce a conflict which must of necessity be reflected in the physical body, producing its own specific type of malady.

'... The result of greed and domination of others is such diseases as will render the sufferer a slave to his own body, with desires and ambitions curbed by the malady.'*

3.   Edward Bach's Approach to Treatment

Bach bases his diagnosis on the law of the Soul, a higher principle of cause, and not, like all other schools of medicine in the Western world, on the limited aspect of personality and the sphere of physical action.

Edward Bach did not use the physical symptoms to make his diagnosis, but solely and entirely the negative soul states that are the consequence of conflict in carrying out the intentions of Soul and Personality and may in the end lead to physical illness.

These negative soul states are not, however, treated as symptoms to be 'fought', for that would maintain them in their energy. Instead, they are flooded, as it were, with higher, harmonious energy waves, so that they 'melt away as snow in the sunshine', as Bach put it. How can we picture this?

---

*Anorexia nervosa in puberty may serve as an example here. Bach would have considered the patient to be the slave of her own body, in this case the slave of her powerful, 'greedy', sexual drive. The illness prevents these desires and drives to be brought to realization, and the illness, i.e. refusal to eat, delays or prevents feminine development.

The flowers used by Bach are from certain plants of a higher order, as he called it. Each embodies a certain soul quality, or, to put it in energetic terms, has a particular energy wavelength. Each of these 'plant-based' soul qualities is in tune with a certain soul quality in a person, i.e. with a certain frequency in the human energy field. The human Soul contains all 38 soul qualities of the Bach Flowers — as energy potentials, virtues, or divine sparks.

When conflict has arisen between the intentions of Soul and of Personality within a certain soul quality or energy potential, the wavelength in the energy field is distorted at that point, it is out of harmony, and slowed down. Such a distortion will have a negative effect on the person's whole psyche, and, as Edward Bach put it, a negative state of mind and soul develops.

How does a Flower Remedy act in such a situation?

The Flower Remedy has the same harmonious energy frequency as the human soul quality concerned, but in this case without distortion and at the normal rhythm. It therefore has an affinity to the human soul quality and is able to establish contact with it, and with its own harmonious frequency waves re-establish harmony in the soul.*

To put it another way: The Bach Flower Remedy acts as a form of catalyst, re-establishing contact between Soul and Personality at the point where this has become broken. The Soul is able to communicate its intentions to the Personality again. Life returns to an area where disharmony and rigidity had taken over. Or, as Bach said: The human being becomes very much himself again at a point where he had ceased to be quite himself.

The Personality, caught up in the confusion and restriction that is only too human, finds a way out again, back to the soul qualities or virtues that give meaning to our existence on this planet and bring harmony.

4. A Simple New Method of Potentization
Plants have been used for medicinal purposes from time immemorial. Bach, however, makes distinction between plants that relieve symptoms and those that contain genuine healing powers. The latter are plants of a 'higher order'. He

---

*Music and colour therapy are based on similar principles.

found them by an intuitive method and called them 'the happy fellows of the plant world'. His sensitivity was so highly developed at that time that he merely had to place a petal from the plant concerned on his tongue to be aware of its effects on body, soul and spirit. It is interesting to note that all the plants are non-toxic, and that many of them do not reveal their quality to the eye. Some of them are also used in another form in herbal medicine, but the majority are simply classified as weeds. It is important to gather them only in places where nature is still unspoilt, where they are growing in the wild. Cultivated, they would lose their healing powers.

The plant itself is not destroyed or damaged. The flower, in which all the essential energies of the plant have concentrated, is picked at the point of full maturity or perfection, that is, when it is about to drop. (There are, however, only a few perfect days when the two essentials, a cloudless sunny sky and full maturity of the flowers, coincide.)

The time interval between the picking of the flowers and their preparation is kept to a minimum so that hardly any energy is lost. The whole is a harmonious process of natural alchemy, involving the tremendous powers of all four elements. Earth and air have brought the plant to the point of ripeness. The sun, or the elements of fire, is used to liberate the soul of the plant from its body. Water finally serves as the vehicle, for a higher purpose.

Edward Bach asked his homoeopathic colleagues: 'Let not the simplicity of this method deter you from its use, for you will find the further your researches advance, the greater you will realize the simplicity of all Creation.'

5. Simplicity as the Basic Principle for the Use of the Flower Remedies

The term 'simplicity' tends to be misunderstood in a world of increasing sophistication, being sometimes equated with 'primitiveness'. Simplicity has to do with unity, perfection and harmony. That is the reason why everybody feels attracted to the 'simple things in life', however vaguely. To perceive the unity and simplicity that lies behind even the greatest differentiation and apparent complexity of a process, it is necessary to have not only objectivity, perceptiveness

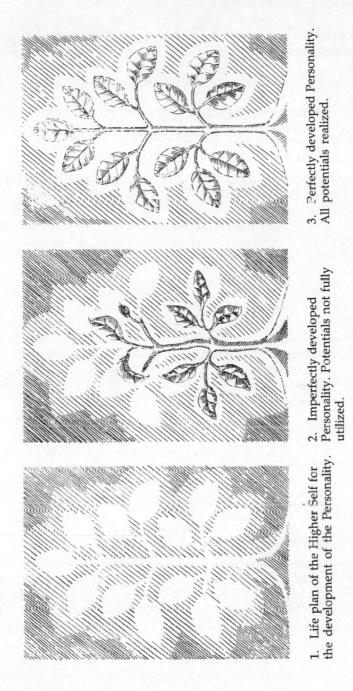

1. Life plan of the Higher Self for the development of the Personality.

2. Imperfectly developed Personality. Potentials not fully utilized.

3. Perfectly developed Personality. All potentials realized.

and the ability to grasp the whole, but also a fundamental readiness to see oneself as part of a whole, a part that in the final instance is governed by a unified, simple creative principle.

It cannot be without reason that practically all the great scientists have at the end of their lives come to accept this view. It is the primary aim and outcome of Bach Flower Therapy to restore and reaffirm this fundamental attitude in every human being.

B. A POSSIBLE PSYCHODYNAMIC INTERPRETATION

Bach practitioners who are particularly interested in psychology put the emphasis on changes in consciousness and the process of psychic development. They run a certain risk at times of getting caught up within the confines of the Personality, and failing to reach the spiritual level of Edward Bach's approach.

Like Edward Bach, they start from the concept of a Higher Self wishing to come to realization through the individual or Personality. The growth process as seen in this interpretation runs in a number of cycles that are different and distinct but also complementary.

Apart from the cycle of physical development that is obvious to everybody, there are also cycles of spiritual and of soul development, to mention just the major ones.

The purpose of life is to pass through all these cycles with increasing awareness, living them through, so that in the course of life the whole potential of the Higher Self may be realized. Anything that will assist this process of conscious realization — even events that initially may appear negative — is considered positive. Anything that darkens consciousness is negative and will sooner or later lead to illness. The key issue in this psychodynamic approach is to aim for and accept constructive change consciously. To illustrate this, here is a greatly simplified example:

The Higher self wishes to express its potential for self-confidence and readiness to accept risk, through the Personality. It sends out appropriate energetic impulses that are received by the 'I' of the Personality. The person gets the idea of opening a flower shop. Using the energy coming in from the Higher self, he or she sets about the realization of the idea with elan, and following the obligatory positive and negative experiences becomes a contented florist.

What has happened? The potential of the Higher Self has found expression in the Personality. The Personality has become enriched.

Unfortunately, the impulses coming from the Higher self cannot always be accepted and realized as simply as that. Very often, the following happens: Painful childhood experiences, faulty upbringing, negative environmental factors etc. make it appear to the individual that the messages from the Higher Self are not acceptable. He attempts to silence these impulses within him, responding with an avoidance reaction such as fear, uncertainty, lack of courage, withdrawal or indecision. The energetic impulse from the Higher Self becomes blocked at that moment. The potential cannot be brought to realization.

To return to our example: The person had the experience of his father's business going bankrupt when he was a child, and reacts with diffidence, perhaps saying to himself: 'I don't think I can run a flower shop. Others may be able to do it, but not me.' The conflict between the impulse from the Higher Self and the avoidance reaction of the individual will not only fail to enrich the Personality, but in fact make it doubly the poorer:

In the first place, part of the potential cannot be realized. As a result, valuable energy is blocked.

In the second place, the inner conflict is daily using up additional psychic energy, energy that does not come from the inexhaustible source of the Higher Self but has to be taken from the resources available to the Personality, as it were, thus depriving other areas where specific actions need to be taken.

The person is now given the Bach Flower Remedy Larch, 'for those who expect failure, who do not consider themselves as good and capable as those around them ...'.

What is the effect? Having the same wavelength as the energy potential of the Higher Self wanting to express itself, it is able to make direct contact with this energy. It washes over the blockage, which is at a lower, disharmonious level of frequency, flooding it with its own higher, harmonious frequency. This, one might say, reinforces the potential of the Higher Self, so that this is now able to take the right measures to dissolve the blockage completely.

In the above example, the individual becomes aware of his negative attitude, his lack of self-confidence, and suddenly begins to see things in another light. He says to himself: 'What happened to my father does not have to happen to me. Why shouldn't I be capable of opening a shop? Others manage to do it. I'll simply have a go. And if it should not work I shall at least have learned a great deal from it.'

Obviously, the process will never be as straightforward as has been depicted here, and there will be hold-ups and regression.

The result, once the blockage has been resolved: The energy of the Higher Self can now be fully utilized by the Personality. At the same time the individual again has the psychic energy at his disposal that previously had to be expended daily to maintain the negative avoidance reaction. The Personality has become doubly enriched.

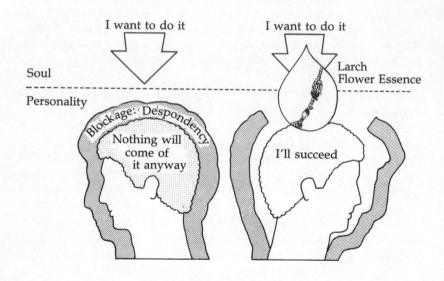

C. FURTHER, ESOTERIC ASPECTS

To begin with, some interesting esoteric concepts concerning the relationship between man and flower.

The flower has always been regarded and used as a symbol

of beauty and the development of highest faculties. Examples are the rose as used by the Rosicrucians and Sufis, and the thousand-petalled lotus in Indian philosophy. The reason is that when man stepped upon the planet earth, to materialize his physical body, the plant had nearly perfected its evolution. Mankind therefore owes much of its own structure to the energies it drew from the plant kingdom, then already perfect within itself, for its own development.

The Tibetan Master Djwal Kul taught* that there is a direct link between man's unconscious and the plant kingdom. Man is therefore able to contact his own essential nature of Higher Self at an unconscious level, through plant nature, and so restore harmony within himself.

This esoteric interpretation of the mode of action throws further light on many things Edward Bach has written in his book *Heal Thyself*. This, as well as the following is based on the work and experience of Ioanna Salayan, using the terminology of Alice Bailey. She interprets man as an energy field with seven distinct levels or planes that influence and complement each other. The only one normally visible to the human eye is the physical body. Each level is at another energy frequency. The six levels not visible to the eye are termed the 'aura'. Practically all occult schools use this concept in some form or other.

At the first, or etheric, level or plane of the aura, energies are collected and distributed from points known as chakras. These are variously related to the other levels of the energy field and rotate at different frequencies which sensitives are able to perceive in the form of different colours. The aura encompasses all levels of consciousness and experience of our Personality. It is governed by our Higher Self. This, however, merely forms the bridge, in the scheme presented here, on the fourth or transpersonal plane, between the mortal Personality and the immortal Soul, the mortal Personality in turn being but one of many forms in which the immortal Soul comes to expression.

The aim of a particular life is for the Higher Self to bring the intentions of the Soul to realization in the Personality. Disease is, according to this interpretation, disharmony or distortion of frequencies within or between different levels of

*As recorded by Alice Bailey.

the aura and the Higher Self. The information pattern of this distortion shows itself at the first, etheric, level, which obeys different laws of time from the physical body, weeks, months, indeed even years before it is manifest in the body.

Some sensitives are able to perceive evidence of such disharmonies in the form of shadows, others experience it as disharmonious radiations. If these disharmonies are corrected at the etheric level, using subtle methods of healing, they will not come to manifestation in the physical body. Ideally speaking, health is perfect harmony and balance between all the energy levels of the aura and the Higher Self.

The esoteric view is that most diseases of modern mankind originate not so much at the mental level (wrong thinking, wrongly understood principles) as at the emotional level, the plane of unconscious emotions and subjective reactions that are either blocked or over-stimulated.

This leads to distortion of energy waves and hence to negative states such as fear, hatred, jealousy, anger, impatience, worry, etc. These first of all act via the etheric plane on the nervous system of the physical body, and later also on other organs.

Today, drugs of all kind, from nicotine, alcohol, hashish and an excess of television to hard rock music and the general flooding with information, are constantly overstimulating us at the emotional level.

Note how consistent and 'progressive' Edward Bach was in addressing his therapy exclusively to these negative emotions.

Is there anything else in this field that could help to deepen our understanding of the way the Bach Flower Remedies work?

Bach said that the Flower Essences establish direct contact with the Higher Self of the Personality and thus become active in all aspects of our nature, in all parts of the aura. The planes of the aura are not subject to the laws of space and time which the physical body has to follow, and incipient illness can therefore be healed even before it shows itself in the physical body. This explains why Edward Bach was again and again making reference to the prophylactic value of his Flower Remedies.

The Bach Flower Remedies enter into direct contact with

the Higher Self of Man. This also explains why they are compatible with practically all other medicaments and treatments, with the actions of the latter limited to particular energy levels, usually that of the physical body. The Bach Flowers act as divine energy impulses, across all energy levels.

Some sensitive healers see or feel enhanced activity within the whole of the aura immediately a patient has taken a Flower Remedy. Many sensitive patients experience an immediate reaction in one particular chakra, and this is on occasion also accompanied by colour sensations. Others have, in double blind trials,* described the particular emotional note addressed by the flower energy.

It has to be stressed, however, that whilst these are interesting observations, they are obviously always wholly subjective. There is no way in which they can be given general application, though some authors are always attempting to do so.

*Neither the person tested nor the one conducting the trial know the type of Flower Essence used in each particular case.

Chapter 3

FINDING THE RIGHT REMEDY

'No science, no knowledge is necessary, apart from the simple methods described herein; and they who will obtain the greatest benefit from this God-sent Gift will be those who keep it pure as it is; free from science, free from theories, for everything in Nature is simple.'

Edward Bach

'Treat the patient, not the disease' is the basic principle of the Bach method. Who is the individual before you, and what is the state of his soul? Life experience and sound common sense should enable us to recognize emotional states such as anger, fear or lack of self-confidence. There is, however, one essential precondition:

A. FIRST SELF-KNOWLEDGE, THEN DIAGNOSIS OF OTHERS

Before we diagnose others we have to achieve self-knowledge. We are only able to understand others in spheres where we understand ourselves. It is also important as far as possible to make sure one is not looking at the other person through the eyes of one's own fears, inhibitions and prejudices.

Experienced Bach therapists always advise, therefore, that at least a year be spent getting to know the Flower Remedies and their effects on oneself, before progressing to the diagnosis of others. A useful way is first of all to go to a Bach practitioner for treatment and observe how oneself experiences the action of the Flower Remedies. How do I feel when I need a particular flower? And how do I feel after taking it?

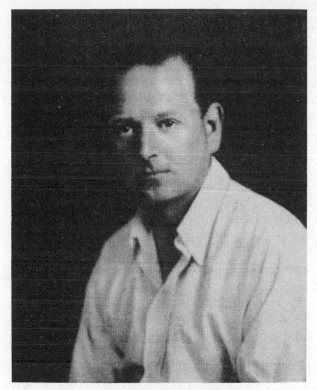

Edward Bach 1886–1936

That is relatively easy if one happens to be in an exceptional emotional state such as bereavement, existential fear, or a crisis of decision. It is more difficult if one's own process of development has no particular highs or lows at the time.

It is a comfort to know that even if one does not get the diagnosis of one's own condition entirely right, no harm will be done. If a flower frequency is not the right one, the Higher Self recognizes it as such and it is not admitted to our energetic system. It will have no effect, therefore, unlike medicaments given in material doses which will always have an effect on the metabolism.

It is also important to keep reminding oneself that the symptom lists given in the following chapters merely indicate trends. We should never allow this to irritate us, but use the lists as a starting point for gaining our own insights into the concrete energetic status that will always be unique.

Experiences Gained with Self-Medication
Work with the Bach Flower Remedies always means setting out on an intensive process of self-discovery.

Often it is exactly the flower with the soul quality we least seem able to relate to that is the one we really need. One has a tendency literally to be blind to certain of one's own character traits.

As one progresses in treating oneself, problems usually begin to show themselves that lie in the border region between consciousness and the subconscious, problems one's life plan determines now have to be recognized and are capable of solution. When this has happened, experience has shown that earlier blockages will then be worked through, in reverse order, right back to childhood. Lesser or major crises of consciousness may develop in the process, and these are sometimes necessary, to set the flow of energy in motion. Many an old problem will once again painfully raise its head, until sufficient drive can be mobilized to effect an inner change. Experience varies in this respect, being highly individual. No two people are the same, and therefore also no two reactions are the same. Everybody experiences the Bach Flowers according to their character.

The intensity of the reaction appears to relate to the degree of sensitivity, one's basic openness to change, and our readiness to take responsibility for our own development, and therefore also for our own state of health.

Some Methods to Achieve More Rapid Familiarization with the Bach Flowers
The Bach Flower Remedies represent thirty-eight archetypal soul states. Julian Barnard* proposes a game that is both entertaining and instructive. He suggests that one considers some of the characters from fairy stories and the remedies they represent. Cinderella, for example, would be Centaury — put upon by all the family and too weak-willed to stand up to them. She never felt herself to be a 'poor victim', and therefore would not need Willow in addition. The step mother was a Chicory type. When Cinderella finally came to marry her prince, her sisters could no doubt have done with a

*Barnard, Julian. *A Guide to the Bach Flower Remedies*. (C.W. Daniel, Saffron Walden, Essex, 1979).

few drops of Holly to overcome their hatred and envy. The classics also provide rich scope for diagnostic practice. What would you prescribe for Hamlet? Most important of all Scleranthus for his indecision ('To be or not to be ...'). Then Mustard for his deep melancholia, and Cherry Plum for incipient madness and thoughts of suicide.

Here is another useful exercise: Look back on your life and identify the emotional states that predominated at different stages. What were you like as a school child, for instance? Were you an Agrimony type, i.e. cheerful on the outside, but 'nobody's business what it looked like inside.' Or were you 'always somewhere else with your thoughts', like Clematis?

Recall past crises, and how your soul responded at the time. Perhaps you almost drowned when small: Star of Bethlehem, and have since been nervous of going in the water: Mimulus. The shock you then experienced may still be present in your energetic system. Now at last it can be resolved. Observe your reactions when you are very tired, are in a crisis, or have to make a difficult decision. On occasions like those you are very close to your own personality, with its weaknesses and negative character traits, and there is no glossing over, no intellectual justification.

Having had personal experience of the blessings the Bach Flower Remedies can give, one may then also consider helping others. Choosing a quiet moment, it is important to ask oneself: Why do I wish to help others? What are my motives? Is it truly only to serve my neighbour? Or what other motives do I have? There may be a desire to shine, to have influence, or a need to make more contacts, or perhaps one has 'found an untapped market'. The more these and other limiting personal motives are to the fore — they are of course always present to some degree — the poorer will be the results in the long run, because one's actions are not guided by the Higher Self in this case, according to spiritual laws.

Work to perfect one's own personality in accord with the divine ordinances therefore must continue to have priority. As Bach said (here paraphrased): The greatest gift we can give to another is to be happy and full of hope ourselves, for in that way we shall pull him up from his depression. In other words, if our own vibrations are in harmony, those of the other person can also become harmonized.

B. DIAGNOSING OTHERS

The ten basic principles, generally known but always worth taking to heart again, are:

1. Before making any diagnosis, consider your own condition. Do not start until you feel yourself to be wholly centred, in contact with your Higher Self.

2. A good diagnosis is never made intellectually. Let yourself become sensitive to the other person and sense the reality that lies behind his words. The work should always be based on the power of love coming from the heart, not the head.

3. In making the diagnosis, you as the therapist are involved in the healing process. Communication always needs to be established between your own Higher Self and the Higher Self of the other person.

4. Consider the other person as a 'fellow human being' and not a 'case'. It needs an atmosphere of complete trust for one person to open up to another.

5. For this reason, include the other as far as possible in the process of diagnosis. Do not proceed on a routine basis. Let the other play a role in setting the key for the diagnosis, letting him choose some remedies for himself if possible.

6. Never be authoritarian. Beware of inner moral judgements. And stop yourself from wanting to be in the right — even unconsciously.

7. The most important goal of Bach therapy is to stimulate the Higher Self of the other person so that it wishes to heal itself. 'Heal Thyself!' Part of this is that the other first of all accepts his condition or illness as a legitimate part of his personality, grasps its meaning, and takes inner responsibility for it, without judging himself. He needs to consciously aim for a change, and know that there will be a change in him.

8. The other person has to become active. He needs to learn

to co-operate with the energy of the Flower Remedy. With your assistance, he should therefore gain access to all desirable information on the principles of the Flower Remedies, their distinction from the usual type of medicament, and also on psychological mechanisms and philosophical aspects.

9. It is always the development of the positive other side of what at present is a negative emotional state that will bring the Higher Self to realization. Talking to the other person, one should aim therefore not so much to dwell on negative symptoms, but to join forces in working out the positive qualities or virtues to be achieved by him. He should not, for instance, go away under the impression that he is too impatient and therefore needs Impatiens. Instead his thoughts should be: 'Impatiens will help me at last to use my superior qualities more meaningfully for myself and my fellow men.'

10. Finally, you as the therapist should be convinced, and with you the person you are treating, that in the final instance, the success of treatment does not lie in our hands.

Diagnosis Based on Dialogue

If the other person does not start to speak of his problems of his own accord, gentle attempts should be made to establish the following:

What is his attitude to life? What is his attitude to himself? What 'adult games' is he playing? His mode of speech and choice of phrase will already provide some important pointers to particular Bach Flower Remedies. Is his delivery rushed, slow or hesitant? Does he speak with conviction (Vervain) or with authority (Vine)? Is he telling his tale in a low, anxious voice (Mimulus)? Does he say: 'I have given up hope of ...' (Gorse), or 'It makes me really nervous that ...' (Impatiens)?

Let us consider further. What can we learn from his life story, his occupation, his family status? What has he been unable to cope with emotionally and physically, e.g. tensions in his childhood home, disappointment in love, drug taking? What is he clinging to? Which of his father's or mother's attitudes and habits still annoys you today?

What situations of which he may be afraid are now imminent, e.g. change of job, divorce, a move to another town?

It is also possible to ask yes-or-no questions on a particular subject. For example: 'How do you like working in a team? Are you nervous? (Mimulus). Do you prefer to work on your own? (Water Violet or Impatiens). The others are usually too slow for you? (Impatiens). Would you try to gain control over the team? (Vine). Are you always the 'fall guy' who gets landed? (Centaury). Or do you tend to button-hole your associates to tell them all about your problems? (Heather).'

Body language will of course also reveal a great deal about a person's emotional state. Is he relaxed or full of tension? Does he restlessly move to and fro on his chair? How does he use his eyes? Is that smile genuine or put on? Does he have worry lines? Where are the points where energy is clearly blocked or dissipated?

In chronic conditions, the healing process can often be set in motion with surprising rapidity if one succeeds, in collaboration with the patient, to discover which unpleasant feeling the other is able to avoid by keeping his illness going. In a case of chronic rheumatism for instance, the following was discovered: The lady felt highly aggressive towards those nearest to her, but did not want to show this. She therefore unconsciously directed these aggressive impulses against herself, developing an illness that caused her pain.

In making the diagnosis, seven or eight flowers may often come to mind. This happens when one has unconsciously been tuning into several levels of the personality. One should then ask oneself the question: 'Which Flowers are needed now, at this moment in time?' It does not always need five or six at once. Often one or two correctly chosen Flower Remedies will prove more effective.

C. SENSITIVE DIAGNOSTIC TECHNIQUES

Some people are able to find the right Bach Remedy by methods that are at the level of physical intuition or sensitivity. These include radiesthesia, psychometry and kinesiology.

Such methods can be a valuable aid in making the diagnosis, providing they are used by experts, and unfortunately that often is not the case. But, and the Bach Centre stresses this, they never can, nor should, take the place of the classical intuitive diagnosis based on talking to the other person.

Again and again, experience has shown that a real knowledge of the Flower Remedies will sooner or later make any form of sensitive diagnostic technique unnecessary. The Higher Self, or intuition, will supply the answers in a flash, before any such technique is even put into operation.

Chapter 4

THE 38 BACH FLOWERS

The descriptions of the 38 Bach Flower Remedies which follow include material from a variety of sources that are currently accessible, but the details given are far from the last word. There is much more to be revealed of the subtleties of the Remedies and their divine healing powers. In fact this marvellous system is only just beginning to show its true potential.

The information on each Flower is presented as follows:

The botanical details have been taken in abridged form from the book *The Bach Flower Remedies* by Nora Weeks and Victor Bullen, who both worked with Edward Bach.

Under the heading 'Principle', a first attempt is made to show the fundamental spiritual quality of the Flower, with special reference to 'misunderstandings' in the development of a person's soul and spirit. This is followed by practical details supplied by practitioners.

The Key Symptoms are the most characteristic symptoms when energy is blocked and the energy of the Flower is needed. They are intended to facilitate a first diagnosis.

The list of Symptoms due to Energy Block should help to confirm the diagnosis. It is based on material from practice records of a number of Bach practitioners and on the existing Bach literature. The intention has been deliberately to list many symptoms, sometimes overlapping, to present a wide spectrum for starting points to be found on an individual basis.

Some may feel that there are negative overtones to the symptoms. Experience has shown that this is how one tends to meet them in practice in subjects who are functioning at a relatively unconscious level. The greater a person's awareness in coming to terms with his own development process, the more subtle will be the levels at which the conditions described occur, and the less will they be immediately apparent to an outsider. It is therefore important not just to take the listed symptoms literally, but consider them as a trend. One's primary concern is to sense and recognize the underlying principle.

For the sake of completeness, it should be noted that a person does not of course have to present all the symptoms listed to indicate a need for a particular Bach Flower Remedy which will be different for every person and every combination of Flower Remedies. If the principle has been correctly diagnosed, one, two or perhaps three symptoms will be all that is required to confirm the diagnosis.

Potential Following Transformation is the most important part of the Flower description. It defines the soul quality, energy potential or virtue a person has and which it is intended to bring to realization. Work with the Bach Flower Remedies can release the negative energy blockage and change it to a state of positive, harmonious flow, achieving transformation and realization.

The Supportive Measures at the end of each section have proved their value in practice for a number of Bach therapists, but are given as suggestions only to round out the picture.

1. AGRIMONY,
Agrimonia eupatoria

Grows to a height of
30–60cm, mainly in fields,
hedgerows and on waste
ground. Flowers
June–August, producing a
tall conical spike of small
yellow flowers. Each
individual flower lasts only
three days.

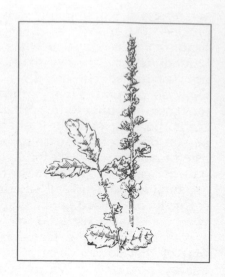

Principle

Agrimony relates to the soul potentials of an ability to
confront others and of joyfulness. In the negative Agrimony
state, efforts are made to ignore the dark side of life, and
there are problems with integrating such experiences into the
personality.

If you call someone who has just lost a major court case and
ask, 'How's things?', you would normally expect to hear
some form of despondency in their response. The Agrimony
subject will in the same situation respond with a routine,
'Fine, thanks', and one will have to know them very well
indeed to sense the underlying disappointment.

Those who need Agrimony always present a cheerful,
carefree face to the world. In practice, therefore, it can be
difficult to diagnose the negative Agrimony state.

People needing Agrimony are inwardly troubled by
anxieties and fears — often material worries concerning
illness, financial losses or problems at work. Yet they would
rather bite off their tongue than let anyone know about it.
The Agrimony person always puts a brave face on things,
and like an actor, will present a cheerful countenance whilst
in the limelight, whatever nastiness may be lurking behind
the scenes.

Agrimony characters have a great desire for harmony and
are also rather sensitive. Discord and tensions among those

around them cause them such distress that they often soft-pedal for the sake of peace, and sometimes even make sacrifices. They are really kind to those around them, in the hope that others will also be kind to them. Spreading cheerfulness all around them they are popular among friends and colleagues, in the pub and in their sports club. They are the life and soul of the party. Even when ill, Agrimony people are still popular, for they play down their problems and their jokes will even cheer up the nursing staff.

If an Agrimony person ever sits down quietly by himself, the problems he normally suppresses will come to the fore. Yet it is not in his nature to acknowledge the presence of problems, particularly any relating to him, and so he will as far as possible avoid being alone. He will throw himself into activities, enterprises and societies, from disco clubs to charitable organizations. Many people with an emphasis on Agrimony also drown their sorrows in a glass of wine, or try to cover up unwelcome feelings with the euphoria obtainable through tablets or drugs. The negative Agrimony state resembles the euphoria produced by alcohol, so that one appears relaxed on the outside, yet there is tension within.

Being very receptive and easily distracted, Agrimony people have no great staying power. A woman who is in a negative Agrimony state, for instance, may be fretting because she is unable to stick to her diet and, driven by restlessness, secretly keeps raiding the fridge at night; this will happen particularly when unpleasant thoughts keep intruding.

In the Agrimony state one will also fret over little things, like having forgotten to make a telephone call, to post a letter, or sexual 'failure'. Many Agrimony types have minor hidden vices.

In the experience of practitioners, a tendency towards the Agrimony state may develop when the childhood home has been much geared to polite society standards, with the children brought up from their early days to 'keep smiling'. Yet disposition probably plays the major role. Compared to others, people with marked Agrimony traits are more focussed on the outer aspect of the personality, not wanting to be aware of, nor to show, what goes on beneath the surface. The surface has to appear perfect, even if chaos may reign beneath.

A person in the Agrimony state reacts like a pair of Siamese twins, identifying himself only with the half of his personality that is cheerful and unproblematical. The other side is consistently overlooked. Attempts are made to pretend to oneself and others that it simply does not exist. In other words: the energy exchange between the levels of experience through thought and experience through feeling is disrupted. There often is a chronic state of war between those two levels.

A personality in the negative Agrimony state is subject to a double error. Refusing to recognize a large part of itself, it is unable to make full contact with its Higher Self and therefore to recognize the programme its soul has drawn up for it. Instead, it acts according to its own limited maxims, and these tend to have a material emphasis. Yet, like every being, it is still striving to attain to an ideal state, and, unable to find this within, looks for it in external circumstances that have a certain lightness. The euphoria induced by wine and drugs appears to come closest to what is desired, though in reality it is far removed from it, achieving not clarity of mind but its opposite, a blurring of the picture.

As soon as the personality acknowledges itself as a unity, and accepts the guidance of its Higher Self, the stabilizing forces of its own soul will come streaming in. It will gain inner strength and sufficient stability to be able to better face the problems of everyday life. Negative experiences no longer need to be suppressed, but can be integrated into consciousness.

In the positive Agrimony state, one is aware of the relative nature of all problems, finding within oneself the radiant, joyful state one has previously been looking for outside. Genuine joy fills the heart, and outstanding character traits such as the ability to discriminate, inner balance, sagacity and diplomatic skill can be put to use, for personal satisfaction and the benefit of others.

In practice, Agrimony is one of the Flower Remedies often indicated with children.

Agrimony children are normally cheerful, sociable, and their tears dry quickly. When they go through developmental phases of inner loneliness and sadness, like all children, Agrimony can help them to communicate more easily what concerns them. It is suggested not to delve too deeply when making the diagnosis for Agrimony subjects, but aim more for a relaxed, sympathetic dialogue.

Amongst other remedies Agrimony has proved valuable in the treatment of addiction, particularly to nicotine and alcohol.

Agrimony Key Symptoms

Attempts are made to conceal torturing thoughts and inner restlessness behind a facade of cheerfulness and freedom from care.

Symptoms Due to Energy Block

- Likes to live in peace, in a good atmosphere; discord and upsets in the surroundings cause mental strain.

- Will do a lot 'just for the sake of peace'.

- Will make almost any sacrifice to maintain peace of mind, within oneself and outside, and to avoid confrontation.

- One's own inner turbulence and restlessness are hidden behind a mask of jocularity and cheerfulness. The motto is: 'always smiling ...'

- Great importance is attached to the impression one is making.

- Problems are minimized and one does not speak about them; they are not even admitted when the subject is brought up by others.

- To escape persistent, worrying thoughts, one is always looking for excitement and variety — cinema, parties, action of any kind.

- Is sociable in order to forget one's own troubles in good company.

- One is a good friend, the peacemaker, the great fellow, the life and soul of every party.

- Resorts to alcohol, tablets, drugs to overcome difficult times and damp down unpleasant thoughts.

- Always has to be on the move, to stop oneself thinking.

- When ill, plays down discomforts; jokes are made even to entertain the nursing staff.

- Secret inner pain and feelings of loneliness in childhood, in children who normally will quickly forget their troubles.

Potential Following Transformation
- Evenness of temper, discernment, objectivity.

- Genuine inner joyfulness.

- The trusting optimist, the clever diplomat, the untiring peacemaker.

- Capable of integrating the less pleasant aspects of life.

- Problems are seen in the right light.

- Able to laugh at one's own worries, being aware of their relative unimportance.

- Aware of unity in diversity.

Supportive Measures
- Take off the rose-pink spectacles and consider situations objectively.

- Consciously register conflicts, analyzing them on paper if necessary, solving them on paper, identifying the underlying principles.

- Try to recognize inner opposites within yourself and relate them.

- Go for depth rather than width.

- Give up stimulants; become less of a taker and more of a giver.

- Do yoga exercises to harmonize the energetic system.

Positive Statements for Practice
'Where there is light, there are also shadows. I am facing facts as they are.'

'I am finding peace within myself.'

'I am even enjoying the darker hours of life.'

'I am establishing links between the different levels of my personality.'

2. ASPEN,
Populus tremula

A slender tree that is found everywhere in England. The pendant male and smaller round female catkins appear in March or April, before the leaves.

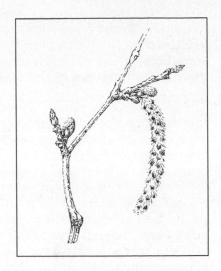

Principle
Aspen is related to the soul potentials of fearlessness, overcoming and resurrection. In the negative Aspen state one is caught up in unconscious anxieties.

It is said that people needing Aspen have been born without a protective skin layer. The definition of their physical reality consciousness from the other planes, particularly the emotional and astral planes, is very finely tuned. These planes harbour not only personal emotional experiences, but also collective concepts such as fairy tale and symbolic ideas, archetypes, superstition, our notions of heaven and hell, and much else. This is the plane through which we must pass every night in our dreams, to reach the transpersonal level of existence where we are able to contact our Higher Self which then lets constructive and healing forces come to us while we are asleep.

People who need Aspen are, much more than other people, flooded day and night with thoughts and images from this astral or emotional plane, without being aware of it. They receive unconscious impulses that their waking consciousness is unable to place, the source of the impulse being unknown. This gives rise to fear. An eerie kind of fear that slowly creeps up one's back, a goose-flesh and hair-raising fear. 'I am so afraid, but don't know what of.' 'I am afraid that something terrible will happen, but I cannot think what it might be.' Those are typical phrases. In extreme cases, the tortures of hell are suffered, and the whole body gets involved, with trembling, bouts of sweating, a fluttery sensation in the stomach. But the fear remains impotent, there is nothing one can do. This is frustrating and leads to even more fear.

It is possible to envisage that Aspen patients get stuck at this point on the fear-haunted astral plane, and are unable to make contact with their Higher Self that would channel helpful forces towards them. Such a state of getting stuck often shows itself as sleep-walking, with talking, or in nightmares. You wake up panic-stricken and are afraid to go back to sleep again.

Children who are more open towards these planes than adults are, often demand that the bedroom door be left open at night when in the Aspen state, or that a light should be kept burning in the room. They are unconsciously afraid that their notion of an 'evil spirit' or 'bogey man' might otherwise become real.

Many Aspen people develop a panic in the dark for which they have no explanation. Some have a nervous, superstitious fascination for occult and magical concepts.

The outward appearance of the aspen tree is a perfect symbol for the extreme sensitivity of the Aspen state. A breath of wind, and the leaves are set rustling. You tremble like an aspen leaf. Aspen people react like a seismograph to the atmosphere in their visible and invisible environment. They have an unconscious antenna for a developing conflict and for psychic currents in others. It can happen that whilst in cheerful company they suddenly feel so unwell, from one minute to the next, that they have to retire. Aspen people register simply everything and this uses up much energy: the office atmosphere full of conflict, the morning rush and exhaustion on a crowded bus, the fear of inflation and war — threats hanging in the air. But in contrast to the Mimulus state, where the fears are clearly defined and can be discussed with others, the Aspen fears remain vague and indefinite. No name can be put to them, and it therefore is difficult to talk about them to others.

Anyone taking Aspen will find the fear and apprehension lessening and inner confidence growing. They will become aware that behind the plane of fear there lies something yet greater and more meaningful in which we are in the final instance embedded and held secure. There is awareness now that behind and above everything there is the great divine law, the divine power of love, making all fear unnecessary. Such trust makes it possible consciously to use the positive side of the Aspen energy. It is the ability to tune to more subtle, non-material planes of consciousness, to explore these planes without fear, experiment with them, and use the knowledge gained for the benefit of one's fellow men. These are the qualities for example of good teachers, psycho-therapists and people working in parapsychology.

Some practitioners specially recommend Aspen in the treatment of alcoholics who are caught up in obsessional ideas, for women who have been raped, and for maltreated children. Such events can be attracted from the astral plane by unconscious programming.

People who have become 'too opened' up by certain group meditation techniques need Aspen, as well as anyone who has been through horror trips due to drugs.

Aspen Key Symptoms
Inexplicable, vague fears, apprehensions, secret fear of some impending evil.

Symptoms Due to Energy Block
- Groundless fear, day and night.

- Sudden anxiety attacks when alone or among people.

- Creepy sensation of fear, as if bewitched.

- Self-deception, delusions.

- Imagination running amok.

- Fearful fascination with occult phenomena, superstitious.

- Fear of persecution, of punishment; fear of an invisible force or power.

- Nightmares, wakes in fear and panic and dares not go back to sleep again.

- Afraid of thoughts and dreams on religious subjects, darkness and death.

- 'Afraid of one's fear', but dare not talk about it with anyone.

- Children: don't want to be alone or sleep in the dark, for fear of the 'bogey man' or similar notions.

- Anxiety attacks with trembling, sweating, gooseflesh.

Potential Following Transformation
- Ability to enter into more subtle planes of consciousness and, as a result, gain insight into esoteric and religious lines of thought.

- Access to higher spiritual spheres. Feels attracted to these spheres and fearlessly sets out to explore them, regardless of possible difficulties.

Supportive Measures
- Hobbies that will 'earth' a person, e.g. pottery, baking bread, gardening.

- Avoid anything that will disturb the mind, e.g. alcohol, excessive exposure to the sun, horror films, etc.

Positive Statements for Practice
'My heart is full of confidence and strength.'

'I am in God's hands.'

'I will be guided, in my own best interests.'

For children: 'I have a guardian angel.'

3. BEECH,
Fagus sylvatica

A handsome tree, reaching a
height of up to 30 metres.
Formerly known as, the
'mother of the wood'. Male
and female flowers develop
on the same tree, flowering
in April or May, as the
leaves come out.

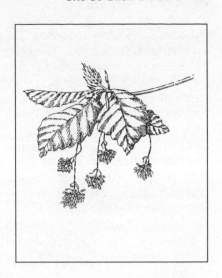

Principle

Beech relates to the soul qualities of sympathy and tolerance.
A person in the negative Beech state will be narrow-minded,
hard and intolerant in their reactions. We all find ourselves,
from time to time, in this negative Beech state, a state in
which one tends to be arrogant and highly critical, judging
others by subjective, often very narrow, standards.

The rather snobbish Professor Higgins in Bernard Shaw's
Pygmalion — wanting to transform the natural, uneducated
flower girl Eliza into a linguistic freak for the sake of a bet — is
an example of the type. Totally lacking in experience and not
having a clue as to the feelings of a woman, he helplessly
asks his friend Pickering: 'Why can a woman not be like a
man?' Having completely suppressed his own feelings, he is
unable to see Eliza's situation, and all he can do is hurt her
feelings with his irony.

Another facet of the negative Beech state may be seen in
the caricature of the strict, pedantic school mistress, dressed
in grey and straight-backed, always demanding absolute
tidiness, accuracy and discipline, having completely lost
sight of the fact that not everybody is born with the same gifts
or has the same start in life as far as social background is
concerned.

The negative Beech state is aptly described by the saying
'sees the speck in another's eye, but not the log in his own.'

In the Beech state, one tends to project too much to the outside, and have extreme difficulty in focusing inward and digesting experiences. Therefore some Beech people tend to have trouble with their digestion.

One often sees the negative Beech state in people from families belonging to a suppressed minority group, having had to swallow much hatred, humiliation, disappointment and injured self-esteem. In an inner process of compensation, the family has deliberately withdrawn into itself and built up its own system of values, which makes them superior to others. Feelings of being denied recognition and of humiliation will then have less impact, being projected onto the outside world in the form of criticism and arrogance. To avoid too much exposure to one's own painful experiences, feelings are as far as possible suppressed, and with that also the possibility of entering into the feelings of others.

Where does the error lie in this case? In its negative Beech state the personality has misunderstood the teaching programme of its soul, refused to accept it, and rejected the negative experiences this would bring. To stay with the above analogy, it has not accepted its role of outsider and sufferer, and failed to cope with the painful experiences of discrimination. Instead, the personality has developed its own code of ethics, incorporating certain defence mechanisms that should help it to shut off the voice of its Higher Self. In our example it develops critical and arrogant attitudes, using them to project unwanted, humiliating feelings onto the outside world.

Such negative projections are harmful not only to the person concerned, but also to the greater unity. The negative thoughts irritate those around them, are projected back onto the personality, and may then show themselves in a wide variety of symptoms of physical irritation. The personality becomes rigid, hardening more and more, having no exchange of energies with its own Higher Self or with the world around it.

As soon as the personality lets go of its limited value judgements and opens up to its Higher Self, higher standards and greater potential for knowledge and self-knowledge are revealed through its soul energies. Restrictive criticism is transformed into understanding, critical sensitivity in relation to others into genuine sensitivity towards the impulses of the Higher Self. Arrogance becomes genuine love and tolerance; the tolerance, as Bach put it, that made Jesus plead for those who had tortured and crucified him, 'Father, forgive them, for they know not what they do.'

There are a number of principles a person inclining towards the negative Beech state might well take to heart. One is the knowledge that each of us is a small cell within a much larger being, and as such only able to truly live by harmonizing with the breathing rhythm and consciousness of this larger being; not by separating from it. It is also important to realize that as a small cell one can only partly understand the laws of the greater being, and therefore we are in no way entitled to apply our own, absolute standards.

Finally it is essential to know that in the final instance we are all only reflections of mutual projections. Therefore, we should not project our own negative apprehensions and defence mechanisms onto other people, but rather try to look within ourselves for the positive projections of others. Instead of feeling cut off, one will then have a feeling of unity, a fellowship of souls and harmony; and this is what a person in the negative Beech state is at heart looking for, despite outward critical attitudes. Becoming aware of this feeling of unity within one, will make the outside world seem suddenly to be more harmonious. Little things will cease to irritate, because we will be more and more able to recognize the unity that lies in variety.

The Beech Flower Remedy helps us to re-establish contact with our Self and with Unity. It loosens the inner rigidity and, as sensitives have stated, brings back joy, cheerfulness and colour to the energetic system. In the positive Beech state one is something of a 'tolerant diagnostician', able to use one's human 'X-ray vision' and excellent judgement constructively, for oneself and for functions in the community.

Differentiating the arrogance of Vine, Beech and Rock Water:

Vine   Inwardly comes into action, wants to prevail, coerces. The underlying negative soul quality is domination.

Beech   Is holding off inwardly, judges, wants to be in

the right. The underlying negative soul quality is intolerance.

Rock Water   Stays out of it inwardly, keeps to himself. The underlying negative soul quality is rigid self-control.

Beech Key Symptoms
Critical attitude, arrogance, intolerance. Criticizing without any understanding of the views and situation of others.

Symptoms Due to Energy Block
- Unable to show understanding or forbearance for the inadequacies of others.

- Unable to enter into the feelings of others, as one's own feelings are blocked.

- Sitting in judgement over others, seeing their faults and condemning them.

- Always sees only what is wrong in a situation, the weaknesses; unable to see the positive results that might come of it.

- Overlooks the fact that everybody does not have the same advantages and potentials, and that everybody can only develop according to their own inner potential.

- Has firm, narrowly defined principles, and inwardly behaves like a severe task-master.

- Reacts meanly, pedantically and in an unwielding fashion at times.

- Small gestures and speech habits of others are trying; the degree of irritation bears no relation to the cause.

- Tensed inside, rigid.

- Being hypercritical, tends to be isolated from one's fellows.

Potential Following Transformation
- Mental acuity, able to grasp the different patterns of human behaviour and individual development.

- Good diagnostic faculties.

- Tolerant and well grounded in life, recognizing unity in diversity.

Supporting Measures
- Be nicer and kinder with yourself, so that you may also be nicer and kinder to others.

- Look for physical ways of balancing that inner rigidity: playful movements, dancing, etc.

Positive Statements for Practice
'I am making peace with myself and others.'

'I am in the other person and he is in me.'

'Behind everything, I discern the positive growth process.'

'I know that I know nothing.'

4. CENTAURY,
Centaurium erythraea
(C. umbellatum)

A very upright annual, between 5 and 35cm in height, growing in dry fields, along roadsides and on waste ground. The small pink flowers form tight stalked clusters at the top of the plant. They appear between June and August, opening only on bright days.

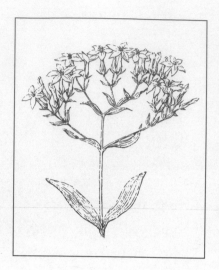

Principle

Centaury relates to the soul qualities of self-determination and self-realization. In the negative Centaury state, the relationship to one's own will is poor.

Children with marked Centaury traits are good-natured, and pleasant, responsive to praise and reproof. They are hardly ever a problem to their parents, except perhaps in so far as they are easily taken advantage of by their fellows and sometimes for no apparent reason become the scapegoat at school. When grown up, they are easily influenced by another, stronger personality who will take advantage of their innately helpful nature, for egotistical purposes. The eldest daughter who does not marry because for years she sacrifices herself to look after her ailing mother, is a Centaury case. So is the son who, for instance, would have liked to have become a teacher, but let himself be persuaded into taking over the family building firm, his father insisting that it should remain in the family (can also be a walnut problem). From our grandparent's generation we know of the pale, unceasingly labouring servant girl who has wholly given up her own life to serve her masters, or the old retainer in the firm whose thoughts, words and gestures are all those of the chairman. Centaury is also to be highly recommended for the young wife who anticipates every wish of her 'mother's boy' of a spoiled husband, wrongly taking this for love, and slavishly suppressing her own real needs at his every whim.

People in the Centaury state often say, helplessly shrugging their shoulders: 'I simply can't refuse him,' or 'I never could say no.' Outsiders often shake their heads on seeing how a Centaury type makes himself or herself a real doormat.

Centaury-governed people will quite often complain of tiredness and overwork, having once again taken on too much in their desire to help. Apart from that, however, they do not find their state a painful one, failing to recognize its full implications, and therefore also failing to notice that with all their service to others they are not fulfilling their own mission in life. The motive behind their helpfulness is nothing but the very human desire for recognition and validation.

In the negative Centaury state, the magnificent virtues of wishing to help, of service and devotion to a cause, show negative distortion. Thus, in error, one uncritically makes oneself subservient to another person and his or her human weaknesses, like an immature child, when one's own soul should be serving higher principles.

In order to be able to serve those higher principles, it is first of all necessary to develop one's own individuality and personality, to make them the instrument of the soul. It is also necessary to know that the personality can only be built up, held together and preserved through one's own will. In the negative Centaury state, an element that tends to be too strong in most other negative soul states — the definition or demarkation of the personality — is too weak.

Some practitioners consider Centaury the most sensitive of all the 38 soul qualities. People with emerging psychic faculties often get in a negative Centaury state initially. A lack of balance will have arisen, with the psychic faculties more strongly developed than the will. In this state, a person is extremely sensitive, particularly to disharmonious energies. They are easily made unsure, upset and hurt. They will often become ill out of the blue, not knowing that it is due to this particular state.

People also easily fall victim to the more powerful spiritual influences when in the negative Centaury state, falling under the spell of 'enlightened' teachers. In the extreme case, they will submissively subject themselves to apparently necessary laws and group rituals, running the risk of completely losing their personality, and with this dissipate their own unique chance of personal development.

Centaury energy will help restore contact with the powers of one's own will, concentrating the energy potentials in the personality and stabilizing them. A sensitive person has described how after the first dose of Centaury a powerful sensation arose, bringing the left and right sides of the body into line and specifically concentrating in the solar plexus and in the thyroid chakras.

In the positive Centaury state, someone is really able to use their great virtues of devotion and service. They are able to serve a good cause according to their own laws, also recognizing the destructive elements to which they have to say no. They integrate well in a group, participating fully, without giving up their own personality. In this way, they are able at times deliberately to make themselves the instrument through which divine powers can stream, for the benefit of major tasks.

Patients in the negative Centaury state should realize, in the course of the therapeutic conversation, that they are not really always helping others by rushing to meet their wishes, but on the contrary are hindering the learning process for both parties. As the saying goes: 'Only a rogue gives more than he owns.'

It is an interesting question to what extent the negative Centaury state does not also represent an 'escape into the other person', in order to evade the process of one's own growing up which among other things also involves having to learn to discriminate and decide.

When the will has grown too weak, after prolonged illness, to do anything for oneself, Centaury will give new vitality to mind and body.

Centaury Key Symptoms
Weak willed, over-reaction to the wishes of others, good nature easily exploited, can't say no.

Symptoms Due to Energy Block
• Passive, weak-willed, guided by others.

• Individuality not well developed.

- Willing, obedient, servile and even subservient.
- Reacting to the wishes of others rather than one's own.
- Allowing oneself to be led astray, in the desire to please, in extreme cases to the point of self-denial.
- Sometimes being a martyr.
- Slave rather than conscious helper.
- Under the yoke or thumb of another, more egotistical personality — parent, life partner, superior, etc.
- Easily persuaded.
- Good nature easily exploited.
- Often a Cinderella for others, or a doormat.
- Unconsciously adopting gestures, phrases and opinions of a stronger personality.
- Easily tired, pale, worn out.
- Avoiding dispute, not standing up for one's interests.
- Tending to give more than one has.
- Easily over-estimating one's resources in eagerness to serve.
- Danger of failing to achieve mission in life.

Potential Following Transformation
- Knows when to say yes, but also able to say no if necessary.
- Able to integrate well in groups etc., but always preserving one's own identity.
- Wisely and unobtrusively giving service, following one's own inner objectives.
- Able to live life in accord with one's true mission.

Supporting Measures
- Before making any decision, ask yourself: 'What do I really want?'

- Any time someone makes a request, ask yourself: 'What are their real motives?'

- Mentally protect the solar plexus, for example, imagining putting on a belt of white light.

Positive Statements for Practice

'I am solely responsible for my development.'

'My task is only to be found within myself.'

'I am discerning more and more clearly.'

'I am safeguarding my personality and standing up for my own needs.'

5. CERATO,
Ceratostigma
willmottiana

A flowering plant from the
Himalayas, about 60cm in
height. It does not grow wild
in England, but is cultivated
in cottage gardens. The pale
blue tubular flowers are
about 1cm in length. They
are gathered in August and
September.

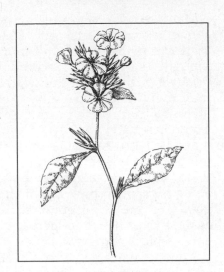

Principle

Cerato relates to the principle of inner certainty, the 'inner voice', intuition. In the negative Cerato state problems arise in accepting one's own correct judgements, without being actually aware of this.

A decision has to be made: the answer comes intuitively, but the head, the rational mind, does not accept this intuitive response, rapidly covering it over with all kinds of routine arguments and adopted behaviour patterns. Something intuitively known to be right cannot be put into practice with conviction. An unconscious conflict arises. It leads to doubt as to the correctness of one's own decisions; failure to trust one's intuition.

The Cerato error consists of the personality refusing to perceive and acknowledge the role of the Higher Self. Instead of realizing that only our Higher Self is able to guide us to what is best in us, the answer is sought in the outside world, often in popular theories, doctrines, and in the experience of people who are quite different from us.

People needing Cerato are constantly getting on the nerves of others with their questions concerning subjective problems and minor issues. 'What would you do if you were in my place? I know perfectly well, of course, but somehow I do not feel I can rely on that. It can't be as simple as that...' — these are typical Cerato phrases.

Many people who are in the Cerato state are not at all aware that, in fact, they know a great deal. They will therefore gather more and more information, hoarding it as though in a savings account instead of working with it. Because of this, their knowledge will not help them to gain their own living experience. Yet certainty and trust in one's own ability to decide can arise only from genuine personal experience.

People who are again and again following current diet fads, unquestioningly, even if they know they will not be good for them, are in the negative Cerato state. 'I know onions don't agree with me, but surely if the diet says so they *have* to be good for me ...' Cerato patients often harm themselves against their better judgement and therefore appear foolish and stupid to others.

Anyone working with Cerato will find the inner voice growing stronger again. And the more one trusts in it, the more clearly it will speak. You will find, to your pleasure, that suddenly all necessary knowledge is at your fingertips just at the right moment, so that you are able to make rapid decisions, diagnoses, interpretations and correlations. A great desire then often arises to share such knowledge with others.

The positive side of the Cerato energy is an attitude of quiet certainty, so that no argument, however convincing it may appear, will deflect one from a decision one has recognized to be the right one.

Practitioners report that the dream life is often greatly stimulated by Cerato, and dreams are remembered better.

The seeds for subsequent Cerato states are often sown during schooldays, when the curriculum is too demanding, suppressing development of intuition in many children.

Cerato Key Symptoms
Lack of confidence in own decisions

Symptoms Due to Energy Block
- Distrusts own judgement.

- Constantly asking others for advice.

- Talks a great deal, getting on the nerves of others by cutting in with questions.

- Excessive thirst for information.

- Knowledge is hoarded but not used.

- Allows oneself to be made unsure by the decisions of others.

- Allows oneself to be led astray against one's own better judgement and to one's own disadvantage.

- Needs the approval of others.

- Opinions uncertain, changeable, vacillating.

- Appears gullible or simple, even stupid.

- Feeling of identity is weak.

- Likes convention, and wants to know what is 'in'.

- Tendency to imitate attitudes of others.

- Poor concentration due to lack of confidence in own judgement.

- Lacking in trust in others, not trusting in own judgement.

Potential Following Transformation
- Intuitive and capable of enthusiasm, curious, eager to learn.

- Able to gather information, organize and use it.

- Happy to pass on knowledge.

- Good co-ordination of abstract and concrete thought.

- Accepts guidance of 'inner voice', trusts in self, and stands by own decisions.

- Acts wisely.

Supportive Measures
- Breathing exercises to make contact with the 'centre' of your being.

- Take up contact with nature; silent meditation in nature.

Positive Statements for Practice
'Inner voice, speak to me. Inner voice, I hear you.'

'I take note of my first impulses.'

'Only I can decide what is right for me.'

'I trust in my inner guidance.'

6. CHERRY PLUM,
Prunus cerasifera

The thornless young shoots of a tree or shrub growing to a height of 3 or 4 metres that is often planted to provide a windbreak in English orchards. The flowers are pure white, slightly larger than those of blackthorn or hawthorn, and open in February to April, before the leaves appear.

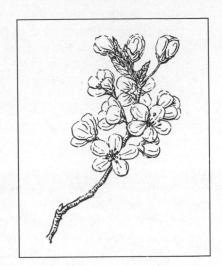

Principle

Cherry Plum relates to the principle of openness and composure. In the negative Cherry Plum state, frantic efforts are made to suppress a process of spiritual and mental growth.

The negative Cherry Plum state is a very extreme one; awareness of it can be either fully conscious or at a half-conscious level. People who are consciously aware of the extreme Cherry Plum state may say, for example, 'I am sitting on a powder keg inside, afraid that it will blow me up at any moment,' or 'To my absolute horror, I find myself having such brutal thoughts as wanting to take a kitchen knife and stick it in my partner's back.'

In the negative Cherry Plum state, people are afraid they may be heading for a breakdown, losing their self-control or even their minds. The nerves are stretched to breaking point; one feels a time bomb ticking away inside. There is the fear that one will be doing something terrible at any moment and that this will be something one will regret for the rest of one's life. Destructive forces are arising within, and it is felt that these can no longer be controlled.

Men who have fought in wars describe negative Cherry Plum states developing after days of continuous shelling in the trenches, or after weeks in a prison camp with vicious interrogations. This reduces the personality to such an extent that there comes a point when it just wants to give up. In the extreme Cherry Plum state there is a real danger of suicide, either physically or at a mental level — which is no less dangerous. Mediaeval paintings such as the *Temptation of St Anthony*, with the powers of hell doing everything to get a saint to capitulate, are symbolic representations of the negative Cherry Plum state.

From the psychological point of view, the negative Cherry Plum state is caused by fear to let-go inside. Efforts are made to prevent pictures arising from the unconscious that one may be unable to deal with. Esoteric teaching speaks of the possibility of negative karmic elements, due to powers having been misused in other forms of existence.

As spiritual development progresses, negative Cherry Plum states may develop before decisive steps are taken. Thoughts of suicide and destructive images force their way into consciousness, though they are not necessarily linked with the extreme feelings described above.

When a person is in the negative Cherry Plum state, the personality has completely turned away from guidance by the Higher Self. It therefore is unable to cope with the more powerful forces it feels arising within itself. It reacts with fear. It fails to realize that there is a law that every mental and spiritual development means activation not only of bright, constructive, positive forces, but also of the other side of the coin, the dark, destructive, negative forces. Anxious efforts are made to keep those dark forces down beneath the surface; but pressure results in counter-pressure.

As soon as the personality submits to the guidance of its Higher Self, it is led through chaos and darkness to the light of its true destiny, and hence to ever greater knowledge. Tremendous energy reserves become accessible. The personality then becomes able to bear extreme external and internal adversities that are powerful enough to break others.

In the positive Cherry Plum state, it is possible to enter deeply into the unconscious and to express and realize the insights gained there in terms of reality. One is able to handle great forces spontaneously and composedly, making enormous strides in development.

In practice, Cherry Plum will sometimes come up even for the first prescription. This reveals the fundamental fear of the personality to open up further to the process of development.

This negative Cherry Plum state is not always easy to diagnose from external appearances. More extreme Cherry Plum states often betray themselves by eyes that are wide open, staring, and blinking less often than normally.

Cherry Plum has often proved useful in the treatment of bed-wetting children. These children are so much under self-control during the day that they can only let their inner anxieties come to free expression by spontaneously passing water at night, when there is no conscious body control.

Cherry Plum may help those liable to commit suicide, particularly people who have been toying with the idea for some time. Here the therapist has to make sure that the patient is also under specialist observation and treatment.

Cherry Plum has provided good support in the rehabilitation of drug addicts.

Differentiating the acute anxiety states of Rock Rose and Cherry Plum:

Rock Rose   Extreme states of terror. These are apparent on the outside.

Cherry Plum Fear of one's own subconscious conflicts is kept inside, as far as possible.

Cherry Plum Key Symptoms
Fear of letting go inside; fear of losing one's mind; fear of loss of control; uncontrolled outbreaks of temper.

Symptoms Due to Energy Block
- Feeling of no longer being able to keep inner control mechanisms going.

- Desperate, about to have a nervous breakdown.

- Afraid one might do something terrible against one's will.

- Contrary to one's normal disposition, brutal impulses come up; afraid of having to do something one would never normally do.

- Afraid of uncontrollable powers of one's own mind and spirit.

- Afraid one is going mad, breaking down, may have to go to an institution.

- Feeling of an inner time bomb ticking away.

- Toying with the idea of putting an end to it.

- Compulsive ideas, delusions.

- Sudden uncontrolled outbreaks of rage, especially in children who'll throw themselves on the ground, hit their head against the wall, etc.

- Parents worried they might hit their children, risk of child abuse.

Potential Following Transformation
- Courage, strength, spontaneity.

- Able to penetrate deeply into subconscious and integrate the insights gained there into one's life.

- Connected to a powerful reservoir of spiritual strength.

- Able to come through the greatest physical and mental torture without 'taking harm in one's soul'.

- Able to gain great spiritual insight, to recognize the true life goal, and make tremendous advances in development.

Supportive Measures
- Find courage to open up and 'take the plunge'.

- Practice plunging also in the physical sense, e.g. from the 3-metre board at the swimming pool.

- Introduce playful elements and spontaneity into your life.

- Yoga exercises to balance the thyroid chakra.

Positive Statements for Practice
'I am dismissing "controlling" concepts.'

'My energy is at my disposal.'

'I accept inner guidance.'

'I am fulfilling my life mission.'

7. CHESTNUT BUD,
Aesculus hippocastanum

The same tree also provides
White Chestnut Essence,
from the flowers, whilst in
the present case it is the
glossy buds which are used,
their resinous outer layer of
14 overlapping scales
enveloping both flower and
leaves.

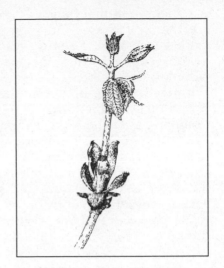

Principle

Chestnut Bud relates to the soul potentials of learning
capacity and of materialization. In the negative Chestnut Bud
state, there are problems in finding the right way to co-
ordinate the inner thought world with physical reality.

A person in the negative Chestnut Bud state tends to repeat
the same mistakes, and in the eyes of those around him never
learns from experience. A woman, for instance, will keep
buying blouses in a certain shade of pink, although she
knows it does not suit her, and probably has five almost
identical blouses hanging in her wardrobe which she never
wears. Asked why she does it, she'll say, somewhat
awkwardly: 'Yes, it's funny really, I keep falling for this
colour ...'

A similar example is of a happy-go-lucky batchelor who has
just broken up with his third girl-friend in the space of a year.
Why, his friends wonder, didn't he just stick with the first
one? 'That's what I ask myself,' he'll say, 'but all my affairs
end the same.'

It is difficult for a person in the negative Chestnut Bud state
to make interim assessments of a situation and really utilize

experiences so that they will profit him in future. Instead, he has the urge to enter into ever new adventures, on a trial and error basis, and the end will almost always be the same. These people are not even particularly unhappy with their situation as a rule.

It may happen, however, that periodic illness develops in the course of life, migraine attacks for instance, always occurring after the same argument on the same subject with the same person. Or a duodenal ulcer that will always make itself felt under the same occupational stresses, punctual as clockwork. 'Whatever shall be', one says in the negative Chestnut Bud state, buying some more pills rather than asking oneself what the connection may be between the duodenal ulcer and one's attitude to the work situation. The thought never occurs to ask one's colleagues what their experiences are, in order to gain new points of view.

A person in the negative Chestnut Bud state is like a show-jumper wearing blinkers, always galloping up to the same fence and again and again failing to clear it, in the same place. From the outside it looks as if the same film sequence were run again and again. There is no progress, no development. The film will continue only once the jockey gets off his horse and considers why he keeps failing at this fence, asking himself where he should make a fundamental change. The moment he has established this, he'll clear the hurdle with ease, and the story of the film can progress.

Outsiders often feel that Chestnut Bud people are trying to escape from themselves, obsessively refusing to face their pasts, and their lives altogether. Being unable to profit from past experience, they find themselves again and again empty-handed. There is nothing on which to base their present decisions, nor have they established any principles on which to build for the future.

It is as if the personality were mistakenly assuming a childish defiance of the Higher Self, refusing to be guided by it, and as though it sometimes would like to play truant from the school of life altogether. Utterly self-willed, it cuts itself off from the actual energetic processes. It is insisting on 'doing its own thing', rather than open up and let itself be carried by the greater energetic process.

When we are in the negative Chestnut Bud state, we need to learn to move ahead with the other fish of our shoal in the river, rather than keep swimming to and fro somewhere in the middle of the river, as though in our own personal aquarium. We need to grasp that we cannot flee from the past into the future, for the future always is merely the mirror of the past, and our real development is taking place now, in the present. We therefore cannot escape the past, it will catch up with us again and again.

Chestnut Bud seems to be a state of very young energy, comparatively speaking, and Chestnut Bud is indeed frequently indicated in the treatment of children.

These children characteristically appear rather absent-minded and inattentive, though they do not let their thoughts dwell on dreams and phantasies the way Clematis children do. They simply do not appear to be able to pay attention. So, in spite of being reminded, they will keep forgetting to take their school lunch, for instance. They will get the same words wrong again and again in a dictation, and fail to keep up with their peers.

Chestnut Bud helps to achieve better co-ordination between inner thought activity and the material situation as it is. Slowly but surely a person learns to consider things quietly, without pressure. He will begin to learn from his own experience and that of others, for the future. He gains distance from himself, and this enables him to see himself the way others see him. On this basis, new things can be learned, and life can be enjoyed again.

Chestnut Bud Key Symptoms
Repeating the same faults over and over again, because experiences are not really digested and not enough is learned from them.

Symptoms Due to Energy Block
- The same mistakes are repeated over and over again, the same arguments, the same accidents, etc.

- Seems very slow to learn from life, be it from lack of interest, indifference, inner haste or lack of observation.

- Does not get enough out of experience, events are not reconsidered at sufficient depth.

- Attempts to forget unpleasant experiences as quickly as possible.

- Prefers to rush into new ventures rather than letting past ones have any real effect.

- Never thinks of learning from the experience of others.

- Seems to be naive, awkward, inattentive.

- Slow learners, mental blocks, retarded development.

- Physical illness appearing regularly, at periodic intervals, without knowing why.

Potential Following Transformation
- Mentally flexible, a good learner.

- Mentally active, also learning by observing the behaviour of others.

- Follows life's events with attention, taking note particularly of all that is negative and of own errors.

- Attention is always focussed on the present, with every experience an inner gain.

- Getting the best out of what daily life has to give.

- Able to see oneself and one's faults from a distance, as others see them.

Supportive Measures
- Every evening review the day that has passed and decide: What new things have I learned: What shall I do different next time, and how?

- Hobbies that will 'earth' a person, gardening, pottery, etc.

Positive Statements for Practice
'I am learning something new from every experience.'

'Earlier and earlier I am realizing what is coming toward me, recognizing possible errors.'

'I see things as they are.'

'Inner calmness is holding me in the present.'

8. CHICORY,
Cichorium intybus

A much-branched perennial, up to 90cm in height, found on gravel, chalky and waste land, and the open borders of roadsides and fields. Only a few of the star-like bright blue flowers open at a time. They are very delicate, fading as soon as they are picked.

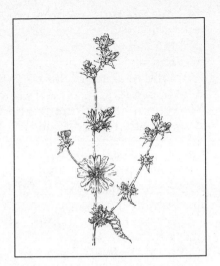

Principle

Chicory relates to the soul potentials of motherliness and selfless love. In the negative Chicory state, these qualities have turned negative, becoming egotistically self-centred.

You are invited to a party, and nine-year-old Gemma opens the door. She looks sweet, with long curls and her first long dress. Charming. The other guests also think so. Gemma basks in her success, acting like a condescending young filmstar. Gradually, however, the guests begin to discuss more adult topics, and that does not seem to suit Gemma. Pretending to top up their drinks, she moves charmingly from group to group, trying to join in their conversation. When it is ten o'clock and her mother thinks it is about time she went to bed, Gemma's composure breaks down. She starts to cry rather noisily, once again attracting general attention. That is the typical behaviour of a Chicory child.

Many children need Chicory. You spot them from the cradle in that they are always demanding attention from the family, with tears of vexation when left alone. Getting bigger and finding that tears no longer get them anywhere, they resort to new tricks. They'll pull out every stop, from flattery to eagerness to help, even falling ill and using minor blackmail: 'I'll do my homework, but only if I don't have to do PT tomorrow.'

Chicory is a negative soul state that cannot be overlooked,

and everybody's energies are sapped. It occurs in both sexes and at all ages, and it is always a matter of gaining influence, making demands, not wanting to let go of ideas, things and feelings.

People who are in the negative Chicory state expect a great deal of others. The classic example is the 'super mother' who holds onto her children with invisible tentacles, traumatizing the weaker-willed for life, all the time concerned about the affairs of her family and of her large circle of acquaintances. She always wants to put her oar in, she organizes, criticizes, marshals and directs like a female martinet. She will always find something to put right, to suggest or to find fault with. Her motto: 'I am only telling you because I mean you well.'

Often incredibly helpful, she almost forces her attentions on the family — and woe if they are not accepted with gratitude. Chicory characters like to have a kind of possessive pride in the feelings and lives of their dear ones.

Chicory mothers really only feel happy when among their loved ones, and grown-up children have to travel long distances on Sundays and holidays so as not to disappoint mother, and if they do try to go against this, there will be such machinations and telephone calls that in the end they will give in.

Not every child finds it easy to free itself from such possessive mother love. Some sons and their families remain under mother's thumb for years and years, failing to achieve important stages in the development of their marital relationship. When a child finally does find the strength to free himself, the Chicory mother will clearly voice her disappointment: 'How can you do this to me, after everything I have done for you', she complains, full of self-pity.

In very extreme cases hysterical symptoms may develop in the negative Chicory state, to gain the attention and affection of those around by force. How does such a regrettably faulty attitude develop?

Behind every Chicory state lies a deep lack of fulfilment, an inner emptiness, often the feeling of being unwanted and never having been properly loved. It is not uncommon for these people to have had a childhood devoid of love. Some describe the feeling as a black hole or a bottomless barrel that has to be filled with affection, recognition and self-assurance over and over again. A powerful will and the whole of one's manipulative skill is used to meet this need in the negative Chicory state. Being unable to give any love oneself in this empty state, there is a feeling of inner uncertainty and fear of all kinds of losses. If feelings are evoked they will often be tied in with a demand such as: 'I love you, on condition that...' An English Bach practitioner aptly described the negative Chicory state as 'the needy mother' (as distinct from Heather, 'the needy child').

Chicory people have the potential for great inner strength and true ability to love, and this can be brought to life if one is prepared to make an inner about-turn. It has to be realized that the black hole can only be filled from the fountain of love that is welling up in one's own heart, flowing from one's own soul without ceasing. As soon as the bidding of the soul is heard and activity is selflessly devoted to the service of others and the greater whole, it will be found that the fountain of divine love begins to flow, and tremendous power and security are arising within. It will then no longer be necessary to gain affection and love by force, they will come of their own accord. Nor is it necessary any longer to fear the loss of such affection, for the inner soul fountain never ceases to flow.

Bach himself compared the positive Chicory state with the archetype of the 'universal mother', the motherly soul potential that lies latent in every human being, both man and woman. Esoteric teachers have put forward the hypothesis that so many people are getting into a negative Chicory state because here, in the West, too many facets of the great archetypal maternal energy have been suppressed, with attention focussed only on the aspect that is the most acceptable, that of the 'virgin', as embodied for instance in the Virgin Mary. Another interesting esoteric thought is that people who during many lives were under the all-encompassing influence of 'mother church' are particularly predestined for negative Chicory states.

In the positive Chicory state, the great maternal energy can be positively brought to fruition, it is possible to draw on rich sources, to give selflessly, not expecting anything in return, not even in one's heart. One is truly dedicated to the interests of others. Wings are spread of warmth, kindness and security, providing shelter for others.

Chicory Key Symptoms

Possessive attitude, excessively interfering and secretly manipulating. Demanding full support from those around, lapsing into self-pity if unable to have one's will.

Symptoms Due to Energy Block

- Egoistic, domineering; demanding a lot, which unnerves others.

- Watching over the needs, wishes and progress of family and circle of friends, like a lesser martinet.

- Takes pleasure in constantly commenting on things, correcting, criticizing.

- Has to have 'loved ones' round one like a court, in order to unobtrusively monitor and direct their lives.

- Does everything for others, almost forcing good deeds on them. Motto: 'you'll have it, even if it kills you!'

- Selfishness, conditional love: 'I do love you, on condition that ...'

- With a certain inner pride of ownership toying with the affection offered by others.

- Manipulates, playing the diplomat, cleverly manages to gain one's will or retain influence.

- Emotional blackmail.

- Wants to hold onto emotional bonds that have had their day, e.g. mother-child relationship, bride and groom situation, etc.

- Finds it hard to forgive and forget.

- Secret fear of losing friends, relationships or possessions.

- Easily feels slighted, passed over or hurt.

- Exaggerates in description of one's 'misery'.

- May escape into illness on occasion, to gain sympathy or achieve ends.

- Grows very angry if not getting one's way, possibly playing the martyr; may break into tears at the ingratitude of others.

- Speaks of 'what the other owes one'.
- Super mothers, firmly holding the reins in the family.
- Children constantly in need of attention, don't like to be on their own, clinging, etc.
- May shy from physical contact with others.

Potential Following Transformation
- 'The eternal mother' (archetype).
- Gives great love and devotion to the care of others.
- Gives without expecting or needing anything in return.
- Warmth, kindness, sensitivity; secure in oneself.
- Gives security and a sense of protection to others.

Supportive Measures
- Physical relaxation exercises.
- Have a massage.
- Breathing exercises to stimulate the heart chakra.

Positive Statements for Practice
'I give undemandingly.'

'I let go what I have been holding on to.'

'I respect the territory of every individual.'

'I am drawing on rich sources.'

'I am finding security within myself.'

'I am opening up to the divine source within me.'

9. CLEMATIS,
Clematis vitalba
(popular name:
traveller's joy)

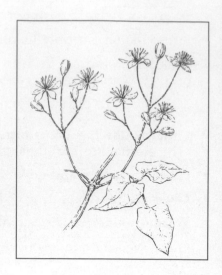

A woody climber found on
chalky soils and limestone,
on embankments, in hedges,
thickets and woodlands. The
stem of an older plant may
be up to 12 metres in length
and is rope-like. Flowering
from July to September. The
fragrant flowers are
surrounded by four greeny
white, downy sepals. In the
autumn, the stamens
develop into long silvery
thread like filaments like an
old man's hair, hence also
the name, old man's beard.

Principle
Clematis relates to the soul potential of creative idealism. In
the negative Clematis state, the personality seeks to take as
little part in real life as possible, withdrawing into its own
world of rich imagination.

You meet your neighbour's little daughter in the street. She
looks at you with large far-away eyes, showing not the least
sign of recognition — typically Clematis. And the nine-year-
old, our little absent-minded professor, is physically with us
at lunch, but in his thoughts he is travelling through space,
the commander of a spaceship. And then there is the violinist
from next door, a lady appearing slightly indifferent and
awkward in everyday life. She, too, is a Clematis person.

'Really? You don't say!' This is the kind of phrase one often
hears from Clematis people, for they are not really interested
in what another wants to tell them, being completely
elsewhere with their thoughts.

People who are in the Clematis state are wanderers
between the worlds. Reality does not hold much attraction
for them, and whenever possible they will withdraw from the
painful present, into their castles in the air. When things

seem to be getting unpleasant, or even difficult, they will often make highly unrealistic suggestions as to a solution, to the horror of their husband or wife, or give themselves up to idealistic illusions.

In the negative Clematis state, the personality apparently attaches little importance to physical reality. This is also why there can be too little energy available at the physical level. A person much in need of Clematis tends to suffer from cold hands and feet, and the head sometimes feels completely empty. Memory can be weak, and details in particular are recalled only with difficulty. He'll dash for the kitchen, bump into the door post because of poor body orientation, and then, in the kitchen, no longer remember what it was he wanted.

Much preferring to run his own 'films' in his 'inner cinema', rather than participate on the great world stage of reality, a Clematis person may possibly sooner or later develop visual or hearing problems. His dreaminess will tend to involve him in traffic accidents. People in the Clematis state like to sleep long and deep, deliberately, and sometimes also inadvertently when watching television, at a lecture or during a sermon. Their lively inner life does not leave much power of concentration for the subject in question. Clematis people nearly always seem a bit sleepy. They are really never wholly awake.

With most of their psychic energy getting used up on inner planes, one will never see a Clematis person become violent. He shows little agression or anxiety. Good news is often received with the same irritating indifference as ill-tidings.

When Clematis people fall ill, the physician has his work cut out, for their instinct for self-preservation is weak and therefore also their desire to get well. Sometimes one almost gets the impression that Clematis patients have no really great objection to departing from this earth, perhaps wishing to be united again with someone they love. Edward Bach called the Clematis state a polite form of suicide. The romantic longing-for-death movement towards the end of the nineteenth century was a perfect example of the negative Clematis state.

Clematis people sometimes prove to have a greater creative potential than the average person. They therefore often follow occupations where dreams are produced, in the fashion trade, film industry and journalism. If their creative potential cannot be brought to realization, a negative Clematis state will almost automatically arise, with creative energy then taking such forms as exaggerated romanticism, eccentricity, and all kinds of delusions.

Many people who are in the negative Clematis state like to express hopes for a better future, when at last the true human ideals will be realized, very much as many people are now waiting for total collapse into chaos, hoping that this will at last be followed by the 'new age', a new millenium.

The problem is that a personality in the negative Clematis state does not consider that the future is always shaped in the present, and that a higher vision has planned this mission to involve every energy, every hand, every head, and every heart. Anyone who simply gets off and waits for the moment to come will not only do harm to the great whole, but also has misunderstood the intention of his own soul and the meaning of his life on earth.

If the personality opens up to its real mission, it will more and more come to see the real connections between the physical and the spiritual world, and the deeper meaning of all that happens. With this, its real life will become more interesting day by day.

The positive Clematis energy may be seen in people who have control of their fertile imagination and are able to bring it to fruition in the material world to good effect, enriching the world around them due to the beauty and sensitivity of their thoughts and actions, as artists, for example, as healers, and as practical idealists.

Clematis may be used as a long-term remedy, but can also be useful with all the passing mental or physical states where joy, sadness or physical circumstances distract consciousness from the present situation.

Typical Clematis people are even less able to tolerate psychotropic drugs, drug experiments and loss of sleep than the average person. Some practitioners use Clematis to avert the threat of infection, because it strengthens the bonds between the physical body and the other levels.

Experience shows that, amongst other flowers Clematis has helped married couples to conceive when there was no organic reason for their childlessness.

Clematis Key Symptoms
Daydreamer; thoughts always elsewhere; little attention for what is going on around him.

Symptoms Due to Energy Block
- Lost in thought, absentminded, rarely fully awake.

- Inattentive, scatterbrained, daydreamer.

- No acute interest in present situation, lives more in own phantasy world.

- 'Wanderer between the worlds', often does not feel at home in reality.

- Idealistic, hoping for a better future; interest in the present only half-hearted, therefore.

- Appears slightly confused, a bit addled.

- Flies into unrealistic and illusory notions when problems come up.

- An unfocused gaze, dreamer's eyes, are typical.

- Appears dreamy and never entirely awake.

- Reacting with the same indifference to good news and bad.

- Hardly any aggression or anxiety, because not wholly in the present.

- Lack of vitality, apathetic, often remarkably pale.

- Easily has cold or 'dead' hands and feet, or empty feeling in head.

- Floating sensation, sometimes feeling dopey, as though anaesthetized.

- Needs a lot of sleep, likes to doze, may nod off at the oddest moments.

- Passes out easily, tendency to faint.

- Poor body image, tends to bump into things.

- Poor memory, no sense for detail, because disinterested and making no effort to listen properly.

- Liable to develop visual or hearing problems, eyes and ears being more attuned to the inside than the outside.

- Shows little desire to get well quickly when ill, physical instinct for self-preservation is weak.

- On occasion would not object to dying, though no active suicidal intentions.

- Imaginative, artistic, romantic, eccentric, but awkward in everyday life.

- Creative gifts not brought to fruition; people with artistic gifts in pedestrian jobs just to earn a living.

- Great feeling for form, colour, sounds and fragrances.

Potential Following Transformation
- Has control of thought world and is daily finding new interest in the real world, because the connections between the different worlds and the deeper meaning behind them is understood and accepted.

- Purposive in bringing creativity to physical realization, as a writer, actor, designer etc.

Supporting Measures
- Creative hobbies to transform unused creative potential into physical form, e.g. weaving, painting.

- Actively concern yourself with the principle 'as within, so without', in both theory and practice.

- Yoga exercises to strengthen the etheric body.

- Much light and sun.

Positive Statements for Practice
'I am more and more perceiving the connections between the inner and the outer world.'

'My mission relates to the concrete here and now.'

'I am bringing my inspirations to realization.'

'I am joining in.'

10. CRAB APPLE,
Malus pumila or *sylvestris*

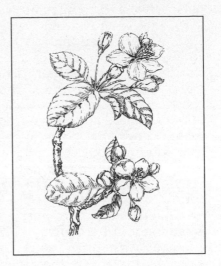

Probably a cultivated apple tree gone wild, spreading crown, short, thorn-like shoots. Maximum height 10 metres. The tree grows in hedgerows, thickets and woodland clearings. The heart-shaped petals are a rich pink on the outside, and white with just a tinge of pink inside. Flowering in May.

Principle

Apple relates to the sphere of order, purity and perfection. Crab Apple often is the state of people who have very definite ideas as to how the world around them, their body and their inner life should be — flawless.

Anything that does not come up to this ideal of personal purity will confuse and upset them. It will make them sad, sometimes desperate, and in the extreme case fill them with self-disgust. This may be a negative thought they had not really wanted to come up, a sharp remark that has slipped out, despite their real inner nature. It may be a harmless little spot on the face that upsets them so much that they really would like to go straight to a skin specialist. Or it may be the inch of wallpaper that is missing in a newly decorated room, so that they can think of nothing else but rushing out to buy another roll of paper, to finish it perfectly. Whichever it may be, it is usually something relatively unimportant compared to the inner energy expended on it.

Again the personality errs by taking the wrong point of view. Details are put under the magnifying glass of one's own limited mental concepts, one gets stuck and lost in detail, finally no longer seeing the wood for the trees. If one were able to take the other point of view and open up, via one's Higher self, to higher principles of order, one would automatically gain distance, to see things in their right perspective and soon be at peace again.

Yet that is easier said than done with people in need of Crab Apple. They tend to be more than usually sensitive, taking in much more, at subtler levels, than their general constitution enables them to cope with. This unconscious stress often gives them the feeling of being unclean, constipated or in need of cleansing. If spiritual means of purification are not known to them, they will try to get rid of these things by physical means. This may often take grotesque forms: constant washing of hands, or taking as many as six showers a day. There have been Crab Apple people who could not kiss unless they first used a mouth spray. In the Crab Apple state, which after all is a misunderstood ideal of purity, the relationship to one's body is often not in harmony.

People who often need Crab Apple are so extremely sensitive that even the tiniest detail will make such an impression that it is all they can do just to cope with this one impression. This leaves no energy for the consideration of wider contexts. Housewives who have the cleaning bug often have the Crab Apple type of problem. Their children's wet feet worry them primarily because of the marks left on the new carpet. The more important point, that wet feet may cause a cold, only comes to mind once the marks have been removed.

The great inner desire for purity will also make many Crab Apple people more than normally nervous of insects, bacteria, food that may have gone off, and all kinds of infection risks. The moment the papers report an influenza epidemic, Crab Apple characters will immediately take every possible precaution, so as to avoid contracting the disease.

That is not as unreasonable as it may sometimes seem to others with a different kind of make-up. Crab Apple people appear to have a special capacity for attracting impurities and dark energies from their environment. Some of them are able to heal and transform such dark forces when in the positive Crab Apple state. A Bach practitioner has aptly called these people 'spiritual vacuum cleaners'. An extreme positive example of the Crab Apple state is the Mahan Tantric, the Master of white Tantric yoga. In his group exercises he will absorb the blocked energies of 150 or more people, transforming them within him, like a filter, and letting them flow back to the group again, freshly cleaned, as it were. He has jokingly referred to himself as a garbage picker.

Such an unusual positive Crab Apple energy may only be embodied in very few people at a time, yet something of this is experienced by everybody who is in the positive Crab Apple state. He will realize that external disharmony is in the final instance always only a reflection of one's own inner imbalance, and that it therefore is in one's own power to make an inner change and in this way also establish harmony outside. This realization is the first step towards recovery.

Crab Apple will remove negative impressions, for instance after a dirty job, after a long and difficult nursing task. Unlike all other Flower Remedies, Crab Apple has a definite double action. Purification is achieved at the mental and the physical level.

For external use, about 10 drops of the prepared medicine* are added to a full bath. Five drops are sufficient for compresses. Crab Apple was often usefully combined with Pine for the treatment of skin problems.

Some practitioners recommend Crab Apple when fasting. Others to overcome the effects of a hangover more quickly — in this case four drops every half hour. Some prescribe Crab Apple for an incipient cold, or to get on top of the side-effects of powerful drug treatments (antibiotics, anaesthetics).

Some Bach practitioners take a combination of Crab Apple and Walnut between sessions, to keep the effect of the other person's energy field on their own to a minimum. Crab Apple is also used in combination with Rescue Remedy to treat pest-infested or repotted plants.

Crab Apple Key Symptoms
Feels unclean, infected; self-disgust. Gets stuck in details.

Symptoms Due to Blocked Energy
- Overemphasis on principle of purity for soul and spirit and/or physically.

- Self-disgust on account of negative thoughts, unkind words spoken, egotistical behaviour towards others.

- Self-condemnation for having done something not in

*See page 207

accord with one's own inner nature.

- Feeling one has to wash away impure thoughts.
- Feels sinful, besmirched.
- Overvalues detail, losing sight of the overall scheme.
- Stuck in detail, letting oneself be tyrannized by minor things.
- Perfect housewife showing pedantic exactitude.
- Everything always has to be neat as a pin.
- Outsiders say, 'she has a bee in her bonnet'.
- Sensitive to lack of order in both public and private life.
- Sometimes has problems with very earthy and physical actions such as breast-feeding and kissing.
- Finds oneself disgusting if one has skin eruptions, sweaty feet, spots, warts etc.
- Anxiety from all forms of dirt, insects, danger of bacteria etc.
- Great need for cleanliness, even compulsive washing.
- Afraid that foods may be bad; afraid of dirty toilets, wrong drugs, environmental pollution etc.
- Great need to exteriorize: nervous cough, chronic cough, chronic cold in the nose, discharge etc.

Potential Following Transformation
- Generous, little things will not upset composure.
- One sees things in their proper perspective.
- A sense for the overall picture.
- Recognizes unresolved issues and is able to transform them.

Supportive Measures
- Accept that man is imperfect.
- Make sure of sufficient sleep and relaxation for the nervous system.

- Yoga and other exercises to clear the glands and harmonize the nervous system.

- Meditation.

Positive Statements for Practice
'Impressions pass through me.'

'I am always keeping the thread.'

'I am a fortunate being with individual qualities.'

'My true core is at peace and inviolable.'

11. ELM,
Ulmus procera

Flowers between February
and April, depending on the
weather, in woodlands and
hedgerows. The small, very
numerous purplish-brown
flowers growing in clusters
open before the leaves.

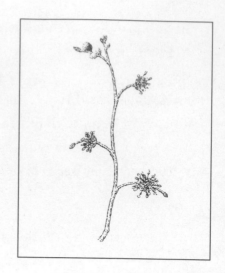

Principle

Elm touches on the principle of responsibility. Unlike many
other Bach Flower Remedies, the Elm energy usually shows
itself in its positive form. In its negative form it reveals itself
as the 'weak moments in the lives of the strong', when
people of above average ability and responsibility suddenly
become so exhausted that they feel no longer up to the task.
The successful owner of a factory employing many people,
for instance, suddenly feels afraid he may be unable to make
a simple business decision, which would have harmful
consequences for the whole workforce. The much admired
mother who is usually so splendidly managing her large
brood, suddenly thinks she won't be able to cope with her
youngest daughter's coming of age party. A capable mayor
no longer feels able to sort out internal party squabbles and
considers resigning his office, although he knows that the
consequences for his borough would be disastrous.

The inability to cope with extreme demands, when
problems appear in distorted perspective, are only
temporary, and the people around feel the world has gone
topsy turvy when their much admired and normally
unshakeable hero suddenly appears small and weak.

Elm characters are of great ability often linked with an
inherent altruism. This will lead to positions of
responsibility, which normally they have the strength to cope

with. But, particularly nowadays, this often means that more and more is put upon their shoulders.

People with the Elm quality fully identify with their task, for the great benefit of everybody else. They do, however, sometimes forget that they, too, are only individuals, with highly personal needs and physical limits. Sudden exhaustion and crisis, the negative Elm state, frequently occurs when increasing professional pressure coincides with a constitutionally determined passive physical phase, e.g. in early menopause. Some time or other even the most powerful motivation will no longer be enough, and the body demands its due. And this weakness causes a temporary fluctuation in self-esteem.

The error is that the person is identifying too strongly with the current role of his personality in such moments, thinking it wrong to follow the guidance of his Higher Self that is calling for moderation. What he is forgetting is that everybody is in the first place responsible to himself, and must first of all meet the demands of his soul, and only then the expectations others may have as to his role.

The weak moments of the Elm type may thus be regarded as warning signals, not to allow oneself to be carried away so much by the ideas and concepts of the personality that the link with the Higher Self is weakened. A human being is able to extend the limits of his capacities for quite a long way, but he cannot go beyond them, as long as he inhabits a human body.

The Elm Flower energy has aptly been termed 'psychological smelling salts'. Elm will lend strength to the strong in moments of weakness. It will rouse them from their dream of impotent inadequacy, making sure they have both feet on the ground of reality again. This will provide clear vision again, to see problems in the proper proportions and be aware of one's capabilities. One knows who one is again, and that one will cope again, on one's own or with the help that will come at the right moment and from the right quarter.

Elm Key Symptoms
Temporary feeling of inadequacy. Overwhelmed by responsibilities.

Symptoms Due to Energy Block

- Suddenly feels overwhelmed by a task.

- Feels that responsibility is getting too much.

- Feeling one does not have the strength to achieve everything one has to and wants to achieve.

- Phases of despondency and exhaustion in strong characters whose normally excellent self-confidence has temporarily disappeared.

- Temporary exhaustion due to constant efforts to perform at optimum level.

- Temporarily doubts his capacities and suitability for a particular function.

- Has the feeling of not being able to keep up.

- Is in a situation where one has become indispensable and now believes one cannot shed the responsibility.

- Too much work and too many different tasks taken on for the moment.

Potential Following Transformation

- Inherent altruism.

- Follows inner calling.

- Above-average gifts, great potential.

- Natural leader, positive.

- Great sense of responsibility.

- Self-assured, confident.

- Responsible, reliable.

- Unshakeable conviction that help will always come at the right moment.

- Ready to attempt the impossible if it is a matter of overcoming difficulties relating to the whole.

- Able to see problems in their proper perspective.

Supportive Measures

- Remember you are an individual person, with

responsibilities also towards yourself.

- In future provide for more breaks when planning work.
- Treat yourself to something now and then.

Positive Statements for Practice
'I am given only as much responsibility as I can carry.'

'I am up to the situation.'

'I always have the help I need.'

12. GENTIAN,
Gentianella amarella
(Autumn Felwort)

A biennial, 15–20cm in
height, growing in dry hilly
pastures, cliffs and dunes.
The numerous flowers range
from crimson to purple in
colour. They are gathered
from August to October.

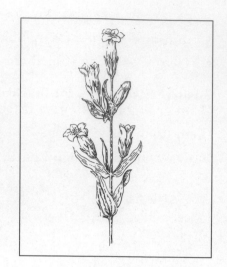

Principle

Gentian is connected with God and with faith. The Bach
Flower Remedy Gentian is related to the concept of faith,
though this should not be taken only in the religious sense. It
may also be faith in the meaning of life, in a higher order, a
certain life principle, or a philosophy.

A person who is often in need of Gentian is someone who
would like to believe but cannot. Where does the error lie? He
is unconsciously refusing to be guided by his Higher Self and
to see himself as part of a greater whole. He is limiting his
perceptions to his own circumscribed personality, cutting
himself off from the spring that is the only source of faith. He
thinks he must grasp everything entirely in his thoughts. He
analyzes, ponders, enquires, and the result of this ceaseless
mental activity usually looks depressing. Unfortunately a
person in the Gentian state does not understand that with
such doubtful expectancy events can but take a doubtful
course. Such an attitude causes harm not only to oneself, but
also to the great whole, but this one is even less able to see.

The eternal pessimist, taking a certain satisfaction in
establishing how badly things are going for him and the
world, the persistent doubter, who does not feel comfortable
unless he is able to worry about something — those are the
extremes of the Gentian state.

As a temporary state, Gentian often takes the form of

despondency or discouragement, e.g. during convalescence. When progress has been good but suddenly there is a relapse, the patient's world collapses and he thinks it will now start all over again.

A typical Gentian patient — and practitioner — will of course also harbour doubt in a corner of his heart as to the efficacy of the Bach Flower Remedies, although he can see that they are effective.

Gentian is very helpful in cases of depressive feelings evoked by a known circumstance. Examples are the death of a marriage partner, continuing unemployment, children torn to and fro between divorced parents, loss of a loved pet, and old people shoved into a home.

Spiritually, the Gentian state may be seen as a blockage in the mental plane. Intellectual powers are strong, but on the wrong tack. A healthy scepticism becomes a compulsive need to question everything. People struggling with philosophical problems, people fighting for faith, are in the negative Gentian state. 'O Lord, help thou my unbelief!' This, the prayer of a christian mystic, puts it exactly.

Gentian helps to build up a faith, not blind faith, but that of a positive sceptic. A person who with the help of Gentian has been reconnected with his Higher Self will be able to see difficulties without falling into despair over them. He will be able to live with conflict, realizing, at least unconsciously, that in terms of the greater whole, conflicts have a necessary function. He will no longer despair on meeting obstacles, being always able to see the light in the darkness.

In practice, Gentian has proved very useful for children who have become nervous and despondent over minor setbacks in class, and do not want to go back to school. Gentian often works wonders when temporary regressions occur in the course of any form of treatment. Above all however, Gentian will help those who cannot get help through psychotherapy.

Gentian Key Symptoms
Sceptical, doubting, pessimistic, easily discouraged.

Symptoms Due to Blocked Energy
• Feels depressed and knows why.

• Sometimes almost appears to enjoy his pessimism.

- Scepticism.

- Doubts are voiced, whatever the situation.

- Uncertainty due to lack of faith and confidence.

- Easily discouraged and disappointed if there are unexpected difficulties.

- Temporary setbacks 'knock one over'.

- Easily feels dejected.

Potential Following Transformation
- Ability to live with conflict.

- Conviction that if one has done one's best there will be no failure.

- Certainty that problems can be overcome.

- Unshakeable confidence, despite difficult circumstances.

- Able to see 'the light in the darkness' and to convey this feeling to others.

Supportive Measures
- Study biographies of great people who had to cope with similar problems and did overcome them.

- Consider the topic of 'how thoughts work'.

Positive Statements for Practice
'Obstacles are chances to learn.'

'I believe in ultimate success.'

'Everything has a deeper meaning.'

13. GORSE,
Ulex europaeus

Grows on stony ground, dry
pasture land and heathlands.
Gorse flowers from February
to June.

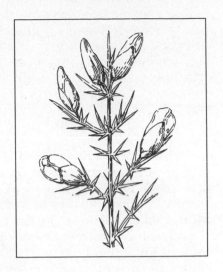

Principle
Gorse embodies the soul quality of hope. In the negative
Gorse state, hope has been given up.

Many people in the negative Gorse state have suffered or
are suffering from chronic diseases. They have had many
treatments, without success, and their doctors have made it
clear to them that they will probably never be wholly well
again. Now they have come to the end of the road in their
minds, and want to give up. For the sake of their families
they will agree to try this or that further method of treatment,
but in their hearts they have long since become convinced
that it is no good.

This mental state is very dangerous, for two reasons.
Firstly, the patient's negative expectations will continuously
reinforce the wrong programming that is the disease,
anchoring it more firmly in the body, so that it can only get
worse. Secondly, the personality is also offering passive
resistance. It is withdrawing more and more from its Higher
Self and active development, becoming more and more of a
living corpse. People in the negative Gorse state sometimes
look like 'basement children', with yellowy or pale waxy
faces and dark shadows under their eyes, not having seen the
sun for a long time. A sensitive has described the negative
Gorse state as one where there seems to be a thick glass pane
between soul and personality; they can still see but cannot
hear each other.

The unconscious error of the personality again lies in a refusal to acknowledge and accept the role of the Higher Self as controller of its destiny. Instead of leaving the responsibility for the whole process to the Higher Self, trustfully going along with it, the personality puts up opposition to the process of development. Because things are not going the way it thought they would, it mentally gets off, never giving a thought to the purpose of the process it has been rejecting.

Such childish attitudes are also reflected in the way many Gorse patients expect that by some miracle everything will come right after all, instead of realizing that recovery can in the final instance always only come from inside. People in the Gorse state will have to learn to come to terms with the destiny aspect of their disease process.

From the esoteric point of view, these people often have a difficult karma that needs to be reformed by suffering in their present life, for the real changes on this planet are achieved through suffering. If such purpose is recognized and accepted, consciously or unconsciously, the whole inner situation will change at a stroke.

A person in the positive Gorse state is able to gain new strength and hope from deep inside, and will then be ready again to follow his own destiny. This does not mean that he expects the impossible — he knows that an amputated leg won't grow again — but he will firmly hope that within the context of his destiny all will in the end turn out right. And so he moves on, despite all that besets him. He learns to bear his sufferings without complaint, having realized that we often learn most through our trials and from painful experience. He thus goes through the further stages of his illness in a state of peace and without feeling hopeless. In the early stages of chronic disease, this profound inner change often is the initial spark that will set a real process of healing in motion.

Very often the negative Gorse state does not appear in the extreme form described above. One recognizes people in whom it is taking a more subtle form from phrases like: 'I have tried everything, but ...' Taking Gorse will in those cases often mark a significant turning point, with the patient entering a new cycle of development.

Practitioners have reported that Gorse will encourage limp plant cuttings to root.

The Gorse state is not always easy to distinguish from the Wild Rose state. A characteristic difference is:

Gorse Can be persuaded to try another approach to treatment even when in despair.

Wild Rose Is even more passive and apathetic. No longer prepared to try anything new.

Gorse Key Symptoms
Hopelessness, utter despair. An 'oh, what's the use?' attitude.

Symptoms Due to Energy Block
- Deep inside, stagnation in the process of coming to terms with one's destiny.

- No longer able to hope for improvement, particularly with prolonged chronic illness.

- In despair, because he has been told nothing more can be done.

- Depressed, resigned, has given up.

- No longer has the energy to have another go.

- Has given up inside, waiting for something to come from outside.

- Allows relatives to persuade one to try other treatments, against own inner conviction, then disappointed when minor setbacks occur.

- Looks pale, dark rings around eyes.

- Has had a long-term chronic illness years ago.

Potential Following Transformation
- Convinced that all will come out right in the end.

- Gains a different attitude to his hopeless position, able to accept his destiny.

- Realizes that hopelessness impedes the healing process and that 'everybody has their burden to carry'.

- Knows that one should never say 'never', and may hope.

- In milder cases: new hope of a cure arises, and this is the first step towards recovery.

Supportive Measures
- Think about the concepts of karma and of suffering.

- Go for a holiday in the sun.

Positive Statements for Practice
'Hope brings healing.'

'Every new day is a new opportunity.'

'I am joining in.'

'Everything evolves according to inherent laws.'

14. HEATHER,
Calluna vulgaris

Not to be confused with the red-flowering Erica species. Flowers July to September, with mauve pink and occasionally white flowers on heathland, dry moors and in open barren places.

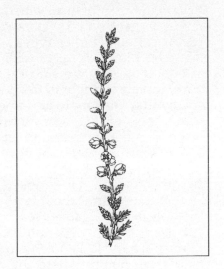

Principle

Heather relates to the soul qualities of empathy and readiness to help. In the negative Heather state, one is only concerned with oneself and one's problems, and even trying to solve them at the cost of others. This state may be of the extrovert or introvert type. Almost everybody will at some time or other be temporarily in the Heather state.

A chronic extroverted Heather state can be something of a joke, and may be defined as: 'He came, saw — and talked!' In extreme cases, there is an almost compulsive need to talk about themselves. They always need an audience, to hear about their terribly important problems or what great things they have done. People in the negative Heather state have the irresistible urge to off-load everything that happens to them by telling it to others. They will monopolize a group conversation, cleverly bringing the topic round to themselves.

Brutal methods are needed to get away from their intense desire to communicate, for a person in the negative Heather state will not easily let go once they have buttonholed you. They will come oppressively close when they talk to you, following as you back away, until your back is to the wall, and if necessary even hold onto your sleeve to detain you. Two other Bach Flower characters are particular victims of this type: Centaury, lacking the will power to get away from its dominant influence, and Mimulus, lacking the courage simply to get up and walk away.

Extroverted Heather types will in extreme cases not even care who they talk to, providing they are able to talk. They will tell their whole medical history, down to the last detail, to a complete stranger in the doctor's waiting room. If there is no one they can talk to at home they'll talk on the 'phone for hours, most of their sentences starting with 'I'.

The 'I' is the focus and pivot of all thought and aspirations in the Heather state. It never occurs to someone in the negative Heather state to take any real interest in the needs of the other person. How does such an extreme form of self-centeredness come about?

People in the negative Heather state have been described as 'the needy child', depending on the attentions and affection of those around it. People who frequently need Heather often come from homes where the atmosphere was cool, so that they have suffered from emotional deprivation from earliest childhood. Lacking the necessary affection and appreciation, the young ego had to fend for itself emotionally. This attitude has persisted into adulthood. The constant talking of a Heather type is in the first place an unconscious ploy used by the personality to make sure and confirm that it actually exists. It can hear itself, others can hear it, therefore it has to exist.

The normal Heather state can be seen in children who are in the ego development phase and exuberantly tell you a lot about themselves. The excessive worrying of a Heather person, his tendency to exaggerate emotions and make mountains out of molehills, finds an explanation in this childhood behaviour.

What could be worse for our needy child than to be left alone by those who provide it with energy? In the negative Heather state, one still lives on the energy of others even in adult life, and therefore being on one's own is the worst thing that can happen.

The sad thing is that others rarely recognize this emotional child state, particularly as Heather types endeavour not to appear in need of help, presenting a masterful and decisive image. As a result, their frantic efforts to gain contact and recognition usually achieve the exact opposite. The enormous pressure they apply automatically makes the people they approach shrink back. The affection that the Heather type is so much longing for is therefore repelled by his own attitude and, although having an audience, he remains lonely inside.

The error in the negative Heather state undoubtedly lies in the personality completely turning away from its Higher Self and the greater unity. It is unable to recognize that there is no need to take by force what will come of its own accord if one allows oneself to be guided by the laws of the Higher Self. People who are in the negative Heather state have to stop being a needy child and grow up to become adults who are also able to give. Once they turn their attention and energies away from themselves and to the world around them and the great whole, cosmic laws come into operation, and the energy, attention, affection and love will be returned to them many times over.

People in the positive Heather state are found to be as good listeners as they were talkers previously. They develop great empathy and, if the situation demands it, are able to be wholly attentive to another person, wholly entering into something that needs to be done. They create an atmosphere of trust and of strength in which others can feel at ease.

The Heather state can take many different forms. If introversion is the keynote, excessive concern over one's own affairs is to the fore. Such a person need not even say much, but the self-centred thoughts that constantly run around in his mind are nevertheless obvious to an outsider.

Everybody goes through the negative Heather state at times when a problem creates such concern that one simply has to let off steam and talk to someone about it.

People gaining first experience in meditation or other forms of spiritual training will often get into the Heather state. So many new aspects of their personality are coming up to face them that they simply have to 'exteriorize' them, in order to organize them.

Superficially, the Heather state may sometimes be confused with the Chicory state when it comes to social attitudes. The differences are:

Chicory   'The needy mother' — wants to hold on to relationships. Gives in order to receive. Self-pity.

Heather   'The needy child' — holds on to those around in order to get a reflection of its ego. Does not give.

Self-centered, but rarely self-pity.

Heather Key Symptoms
Self-centered, obsessed with own troubles and affairs, constantly needs an audience, 'the needy child'.

Symptoms Due to Energy Block
- Thoughts entirely centered on personal problems, takes himself terribly seriously, 'talkative hypochondriac'.

- Wants to hold centre of attention, almost compulsively needs an audience.

- Takes over the conversation and immediately turns it to herself.

- Buttonholes others in his desire to make his point, holds onto sleeves, won't let go.

- Saps the strength of others with incessant talk, a strain on their nerves and manners.

- Needs his fellow men, living on their energies.

- Can't be alone.

- Tends to exaggerate emotionally, making mountains out of molehills.

- Self-absorbed, self-concerned.

- Poor listener.

- Often from a home lacking in warmth, emotionally undernourished as a child.

- Often in the early stages of spiritual development, when one is faced with one's ego and needs to exteriorize many inner experiences.

Potential Following Transformation
- The sympathetic adult, great empathy.

- Good listener, interested partner in discussion.

- Able to enter completely into the concerns of another or something that needs to be done.

- Radiates strength and confidence.

Supportive Measures
- Always visualize the aura of the other, as something not to be penetrated.

- Practise listening; for once consciously wait to see what comes up of its own accord.

- Become engaged in group projects: neighbourhood help, community politics etc.

Positive Statements for Practice
'I give and I also shall be given.'

'Whatever is right for me, will come to me.'

'I am secure within myself.'

'I am flowing in the stream of divine energy.'

15. HOLLY,
Ilex aquifolium

A tree or shrub with glossy
evergreen leaves and brilliant
red berries, growing in
woodlands and hedgerows.
The male and female flowers
are white, slightly fragrant,
usually grow on different
trees and open in May and
June.

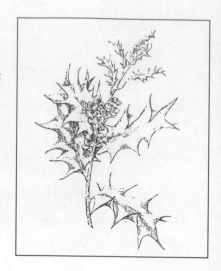

Principle

Its name sounding almost the same as 'holy', the holly is
brought indoors at Christmas in English-speaking countries
to symbolize the birth of Christ. This is no mere coincidence.
The Holly Flower Remedy embodies the principle of divine,
all-encompassing love, the love that maintains this world and
is greater than human reason. This love, this highest energy
quality, through which and in which we all live, is our true
life elixir, the greatest healing power, and the strongest
motive force. Holly therefore holds a central position among
the 38 Bach Flower Remedies.

If this great power of love fails to gain acceptance it will
turn into its opposite: negation, separation and hatred. That
is the most profound cause of all other negative events in life.
Everyone living on this earth will sooner or later have to
come to terms with this central issue for humanity,
consciously or unconsciously.

Going with the stream of love, living 'in a state of grace',
one's heart is open, and all men are seen as brothers. Having
dropped out of the stream of love, the heart hardens, and one
finds oneself painfully isolated, cut off and separate from
everything. Yet the desire for this love is programmed into
every cell of our being, and in the negative Holly state one is
therefore fighting for existence in one's heart. Every being
wants to give love and receive love when born into this

world. If it is denied this, it will experience unbelievable disappointment and begin to delimit itself from something in which it apparently is not to have a part, and to defend itself.

Love being such a tremendous power, its shadow side also comes to expression in enormously powerful feelings: jealousy, revenge, hatred, envy, resentment, malice. These feelings, and none of us is entirely free of them, either come out into the open or continue at more unconscious levels, when they may form the emotional basis for serious diseases.

This, then, is a particular reason why we need to recognize and acknowledge these profoundly human negative feelings in ourselves, for they mirror our innermost needs. They show what we do not have but dearly would like to have, and so provide an opportunity to make the right efforts to attain it.

Envy for instance is a feeling that is widespread today, not only in the business world, but also in so-called spiritual circles. Secretly, one wonders how far the other has got, whether he has already 'reached a higher stage'. People who have entered on the spiritual path have a particular need for love and being able to open up, and such feelings will of necessity arise, until at last the step is taken from separatedness to unity, and we have found God in our own hearts.

The morbid jealousy that keenly looks for anything that will cause suffering is the classical, tragic example of the desire for love in a negative key. Someone who is isolated in his heart and has turned away from love, and now has found another towards whom his desire for love can be directed, will feel himself constantly in danger of losing this love, for, having no knowledge of love himself, he is unable to let it flow forth. Instead, he radiates uncertainty and his fears, and as a logical result finds pain.

It is not only the jealous who need to recognize that love focused wholly on another human being cannot in the long run gain fulfilment, unless it is at the same time, and as a primary aim, also looking for divine unity as its goal.

In the case of jealousy, distinction needs to be made between the morbid and the 'normal' forms. The latter will temporarily arise in any loving relationship. When the highest feelings of love are activated the counterpart will inevitably also be activated, a law that provides the impetus for a further step in development.

We should develop a keen ear for people who say they are so tolerant that they know no jealousy. It is highly improbable that this is a serene, wise person. One would rather suspect that he has already gone so far towards death in his heart that he no longer is able to suffer and to love.

From this point of view it is always reason for rejoicing when Holly comes up in the diagnosis, for it shows that there is a potential in this essential point that is still capable of development, for the person is longing for love and will also be able to give love.

Edward Bach said: 'Holly protects us from everything that is not Universal Love. Holly opens the heart and unites us with Divine Love.' We develop a feeling for our origins, for where we belong, and that we are all children of love. Holly helps us again and again to live in the state of love, in that state of beauty, solemnity and fulfilment where one is one heart and one soul with the world, and is able to recognize and acknowledge everything as part of the natural God-given order; where one is able to join in the pleasure of others without envy, even whilst one may be having problems oneself.

The soul quality of Holly is the ideal human state, the goal we are striving for in life.

'To experience and love the god of beauty and goodness even in what is ugly and in what is evil, and to long, in extreme love, to heal it of its ugliness and its evil, that is true virtue and morality.' (Sri Aurobindo).

In practice, the negative Holly state is often not so much to the fore. One would hardly expect anything else in countries where for generations it has not been considered good manners to speak about your feelings. It is necessary, therefore, to try to sense the negative Holly state of another in the diagnostic dialogue. People who are on the spiritual path need Holly more often than one would think. Holly can be an absolute blessing in the terminal stages of chronic diseases.

In diagnosis, Holly and Wild Oat may be used to open up a case and clarify the situation. When there has been no response to the Flower Remedies prescribed, or when it seems difficult to decide which of the many soul qualities that have shown themselves is the more important, it is best to give Holly or Wild Oat first. Holly is used for people who are active and energetic, Wild Oat for the rather low-key, passive type of person.

A common experience with Holly: When the second child is born, the first often shows jealousy, in the form of moodiness, rebelliousness, etc. Holly has proved very useful in such cases. Also with dogs showing jealousy when suddenly confronted with a baby in the family.

Sometimes distinction has to be made between Holly and Chicory:

Holly   Embodies the more universal aspect of love. Feelings are more painful, and may relate not only to people but also to ideas.

Chicory Embodies one particular aspect of love only, that of giving and taking. A possessive, demanding attitude to others predominates.

Holly Key Symptoms
Jealousy, distrust, feelings of hatred and envy at all levels.

Symptoms Due to Blocked Energies
* Heart is hardened.

* Is discontented, unhappy, frustrated, but does not always know why.

* Feelings of envy and hatred.

* Jealousy, distrust, revengefulness.

* Malice.

* Fears one is being deceived.

* Misunderstandings; complains about others.

* Suspects a negative aspect to many things.

* Easily suspicious of others.

* Frequently feels hurt or injured.

* Is supersensitive to real or imagined slights.

* Belittles others in his heart.

* Rage, anger, violent bouts of ill-humour that may find physical expression (often in children).

Potential Following Transformation
- Living in inner harmony, radiating love.

- Profound understanding of human emotions.

- Able to take pleasure in achievements and successes of others, even if having problems oneself.

- Has a sense for the scheme of things, and is able to acknowledge every person in his right place.

Supportive Measures
- Yoga exercises to stimulate the heart chakra.

- Group work of all types.

- Fall in love.

Positive Statements for Practice
'I love and am loved.'

'I am part of the whole.'

'I open my heart.'

16. HONEYSUCKLE,
Lonicera caprifolium

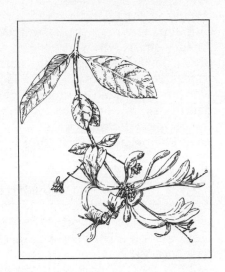

A vigorous, fragrant climber found in woodlands, on the edges of forests and on heathland. The petals, reddish outside and white inside, turn yellow on pollination. Less common than the yellow-flowering honeysuckle, it flowers from June to August.

Principle

Honeysuckle touches on the principle of capacity for change and ability to establish links. In the negative Honeysuckle state, the connection with the current of life is poor.

The problem in this case lies in lack of inner mobility. There is a certain inertia; one is mentally lingering in the wrong place at the wrong time, and therefore unable to act. The classic example is the story of Lot's wife who was turned into a pillar of salt, having disregarded the words of her guiding angel, letting herself be drawn by the past and turning to face back towards Sodom, instead of concentrating all her energies on the present, on her flight and escape.

A person who is in the honeysuckle state lives mentally largely in the past. To bridge the gulf with the present requires a great deal of psychic energy.

In the negative Honeysuckle state the personality refuses to be guided by its Higher Self, according to the laws of its soul, even if it may not always understand those laws. It ignores the fact that one of the most important life principles is constant change, that everything is in a state of flux. Instead, it wants to determine its own destiny, particularly where emotional experience is concerned. The standards it applies in this case are self-centered and therefore narrow.

The widow who for years keeps her dead husband's study so that it looks as if he's just this moment left his desk, is in

the Honeysuckle state. An even more extreme example is the
film actress who has not budged from her days of greatness.
At fifty she is still wearing the frocks, hairstyle and make-up
of the 'sweet young thing', the role that once made her so
successful. Others needing Honeysuckle are the young
woman not making a new relationship after her fiancé's
death, and the homesick development engineer in Africa. Or
the couple who had to move to another part of town and now
keep saying how much they miss their old area. No wonder
that they cannot settle properly or make new friends with
such an attitude.

Such people unconsciously refuse to see and accept new
developments. Honeysuckle types will start their sentences
with 'I used to ...' and 'When I was still ...' more often than
other people. This shows that they are still clinging to the
past, not yet having properly digested it. They are unable to
make a live connection between the past and their present
situation, because they cannot or will not consider the past
from all angles. They fix their mind on just one aspect,
usually a pleasant one. The result is that their bad
experiences cannot be integrated and no profit can be drawn
from them for the further development of the personality.

The Honeysuckle state is understandable, and in a way
normal, in the elderly when they are in the process of
'settling their inner accounts'. Particularly today, when old
people are systematically shut off from the active stream of
life, one can understand they withdraw in their minds to
dwell on bygone better days. The Honeysuckle state
encompasses regret for missed opportunities, missed
chances and unfulfilled hopes. Honeysuckle helps the dying
to 'let go' more easily.

About Honeysuckle Bach wrote: 'This is the remedy to
remove from the mind the regrets and sorrows of the past, to
counteract all influences, all wishes and desires of the past
and to bring us back to the present.'

In the transformed Honeysuckle state one has a living
connection to one's past, learning from it, but not clinging to
it unnecessarily. One is able to work with one's past.
Archaeologists, historians and dealers in antiquities are in a
positive Honeysuckle state from this point of view. In group
psychology or reincarnation therapy, Honeysuckle can help
to establish the link between past and present, and make sure

that the past is given its proper value.

The negative Honeysuckle state has usually built up over quite a period; though it may also be of short duration, especially in children. Honeysuckle has often helped homesick children at boarding school.

Interestingly, Honeysuckle may be used to combat regret that one is getting old. There is a beautician who even puts some drops of Honeysuckle into her face lotion. The psychological state of regret accelerates the ageing of the skin, and such a basic negative attitude finds expression first of all in the bearing of a person, and finally in the tone of the skin.

The Honeysuckle state is in some respects very similar to the Clematis state. Both have the feature that the person has no interest in the present and is not living in the here and now. The difference is:

Honeysuckle	Escapes to the past and expects nothing positive from present and future.
Clematis	Escapes from the present into fantasy life, hoping for a better future.

On occasion, distinction also has to be made between Honeysuckle and Pine:

Honeysuckle	Wistful regret.
Pine	Genuine guilt feelings.

Honeysuckle Key Symptoms
Longing for the past; regrets over the past; not living in the present.

Symptoms Due to Energy Block
* Constantly referring to the past, in one's mind and in conversation with others.

* Glorifying the past, expecting it to return.

* Wistfully thinks back to the good old days.

* Cannot get over the loss of a person one loved (parent, child, spouse).

* Sometimes: recollections of childhood are unusually poor

* Cannot forget a certain event in the past.

* Homesickness.

* Sorry to have missed an opportunity or that a dream remains unfulfilled.

- Longs to be able to begin again.

Potential Following Transformation
- Has a living relationship to the past, but is living in the present.

- Has learned from past experience, but does not cling to it.

- Able to preserve what was beautiful in the past for the present.

- Able to bring the past back to life (e.g. as a writer, archaeologist, historian).

Supportive Measures
- Assume new responsibilities (e.g. a pet, the upkeep of a garden, honorary office in a local association.)

- Occupy yourself with the problems of the present.

- Artistic hobbies (e.g. dance, singing, music.)

Positive Statements for Practice
'Nothing ever remains the same.'

'Life is happening now.'

'Every day is new and exciting.'

'I am identifying myself with my present tasks.'

17. HORNBEAM,
Carpinus betulus

A tree superficially similar to
the beech but smaller and
greener, growing singly or in
groups in woods and
coppices. The pendant male
and upright female flowers
are a greeny-brown and
open in April or May.

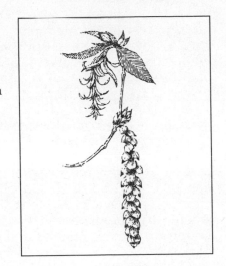

Principle
Hornbeam is connected with the soul potential of inner
vitality and freshness of mind. In the negative Hornbeam
state, one feels great weariness and exhaustion, though this
is largely in the mind.

Every office worker knows the feeling when the alarm clock
rings on Monday morning and dull routine once again
beckons. What lies ahead is a largely familiar, monotonous
working week offering little genuine responsibility but many
demands. A thousand little things that have to be kept track
of, routines to be maintained, things not dealt with. All this is
looming up before one like a dark mountain and one feels
one does not have the strength to cope; although one usually
does.

The Hornbeam weariness is a state of exhaustion arising
from one-sided demands on the mental plane, with nothing
to make up for it in other planes. It may be a temporary state,
but can also become chronic. Temporary, for instance, when
a student has been swotting for months before an
examination, or when a patient has spent a long time in bed
with a broken limb, doing a lot of reading, thinking and
planning. A kind of head-heavy weariness leads him to think
that he is not yet fit to do physical exercises.

The more long-term Hornbeam weariness is characteristic
of the affluent modern citizen who consumes too much and

produces too little. He takes in many more impressions than he is able to digest mentally, and with heavy head finds it hard to get up in the mornings. He lives a standardized life, with even leisure and holidays following the set pattern and often seeming more of a duty. Outside events may be relatively many, but inwardly too little is happening.

Interestingly, the Hornbeam weariness disappears instantly when something out of the ordinary happens, challenging the person at another level, pulling him out of his mental rut.

The error with the negative Hornbeam state lies in self-imposed limits on the personality, often with a materialistic bias. The personality is 'short-sighted' and 'hard of hearing' where the impulses of the Higher Self are concerned, preferring to settle on the familiar automatic patterns. It thus deprives itself increasingly of opportunities for development and everything that really makes life vital and worth living.

In the negative Hornbeam state the energy system of a person has been upset by one-sided demands on the mental plane and too little being asked on other planes. The different planes do not communicate sufficiently, energy exchange is disrupted, and energy conversion reduced. The only possible outcome is an energy deficit.

Sensitives describe the Hornbeam Flower energies as a refreshing cool shower, with the individual energy levels becoming equalized again, given a tonic. It has been said that Hornbeam 'stiffens the spine'. The head becomes clear, perceptions more lively, the impulses of the Higher Self get through again. The right way to alternate between activity and passivity is rediscovered. Life and work become a pleasure again, and the certainty is gained that one will have the necessary strength to achieve what one wishes to achieve.

Hornbeam rarely comes up on its own in a diagnosis. It is often combined with Olive, Gentian or White Chestnut. Some practitioners recommend Hornbeam in compresses for tired and irritated eyes, others to strengthen varicose veins. The tonic effect on the energies has proved helpful in drug rehabilitation. Finally, Hornbeam is another of the Flower Remedies that gives new vigour to limp plants.

Differentiation between the Hornbeam and the Olive weariness:

Hornbeam Weariness due to one-sided lifestyle, mainly on mental plane.

Olive Genuine exhaustion, due to being totally spent on several planes.

Hornbeam Key Symptoms

Weariness; mental exhaustion, either temporary or prolonged, procrastination.

Symptoms Due to Energy Block

- Heavy-headed, tired and exhausted.

- Mental hangover, 'Monday morning feeling'.

- Head aching after watching too much television, too much reading, too much studying and other excessive demands on the senses.

- Feels deprived of vigour; mental block.

- On waking, doubts if the day's chores can be coped with; but this gets better once one gets going.

- Exhausted at the thought of having to face another grey week.

- After prolonged illness: slow to recover the will to return to work.

- Believes it is impossible to start work without stimulants such as coffee, tea, or some form of tonic.

- Comes to life when something unexpectedly interesting occurs.

- Life is too fully organized and has too much routine.

- Get up more tired in the morning than on going to bed.

- Pressure or burning sensation in or around the eyes.

- Often connective tissue degeneration.

- Exhaustion through years of one-sided lifestyle, sedentary occupation, too little exercise.

Potential Following Transformation

- Lively mind, clear, cool head, likes variety.

- Sure one will be able to master the tasks ahead, even if they appear to be beyond one's powers.

Supportive Measures
- Break the routine.

- Provide for compensatory physical activity, but don't set high goals.

- Spontaneously follow up sudden notions.

- Change of scenery.

Positive Statements for Practice
'I feel awake and fresh.'

'I'll follow my spontaneous impulses.'

'I do whatever gives me pleasure. And whatever I do gives me pleasure.'

18. IMPATIENS,
*Impatiens glandulifera
(I. roylei)*

A fleshy annual, up to
180cm in height, growing on
river and canal banks and in
damp, low ground. Flowers
are crimson to reddish
mauve and appear between
July and September.

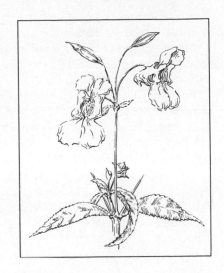

Principle

Impatiens relates to the soul qualities of patience and
gentleness. In the negative Impatiens state, we are impatient,
inner tension tending to make us irritable towards others.

Being quick-thinking, everybody else seems very slow.
One feels like a thoroughbred forced to pull a plough in
harness with a farm horse. Feeling frustrated inside, one
nevertheless adapts to the slower pace of life and work of
others. This adaptation to a lower energy level takes a great
deal of energy, however, leading to constant mental tension.

Impatiens people are not always popular as superiors, for
they know how to do everything better themselves and are
not exactly diplomatic in letting inferiors know this: 'Never
mind, leave it. Before I explain the whole thing to you, I'll
have done it myself.' Instructors of the Impatiens type find it
very difficult to stand patiently by watching the awkward
first attempts of their trainees.

It is unwise to make any critical comment to someone in the
Impatiens state, however diplomatically. They are likely to
flare up, though their anger will pass just as quickly as it
arose. Impatiens bosses tend to 'push' their staff to the point
where they become referred to as slave-drivers.

The regrettable fact is that Impatiens people do not assume
this role gladly. They have no ambitions to lead — unlike
Vine, for instance — and would prefer to work entirely by

themselves and get things done at their own pace, without outside interference. Their independence is most dear to them. Impatiens types know their difficulties and when in an equable state of mind are open to and grateful for good advice.

People in the negative Impatiens state have more active minds than average. They see things more quickly, deliver sentences with machine-gun rapidity, react in a flash, make ad hoc decisions — and will then of course also be worn out more quickly.

The blowing-hot-and-cold disposition is often also apparent on the outside. Impatiens types may go red all of a sudden and just as quickly grow pale again. Great inner restlessness can also make Impatiens people impetuous and therefore accident prone. Yet in the end they have fewer accidents than one might expect, because they are able to react in a flash and therefore get out of many a critical situation.

The error of the negative Impatiens state lies in excessive self-willedness and self-imposed limits on the personality. It is forgotten that every person is part of a great whole and that in the final instance we all depend on each other, including those who seem less capable, and vice versa. Nor does the personality consider that anyone more capable is indeed required to place his greater gifts at the service of others, to help them in their development. Impatiens people have to learn to do what is hardest for them: to hold back from active involvement, to let things happen, to practice patience. This will be easier if they operate not from their powerful mental plane, but think with their hearts.

Positive Impatiens types show great empathy, delicacy of feeling and angelic patience. They fully understand the different nature of others, and are diplomatic in putting their quickness of mind, power of decision and intelligence at the service of others.

In practice, Impatiens has also proved very useful in daily family life. Children squabbling when taken shopping or on a visit, getting into temper tantrums, will respond well and quickly to Impatiens, and so will parents who at times are quick to run out of patience with their offspring.

The Impatiens state is usually very obvious, for these people are naturally extrovert. If they do not reveal their state in words, they will frequently do so in gestures: nervously drumming their fingers on the table, for instance. When gestures also do not reveal the state, then it may sometimes be indicated by nervous skin rashes, skin irritation, etc. Suppressed even further, the state will, on rare occasions, show itself in its polar opposite — extreme indolence and lack of initiative. Children with strong Impatiens traits should be guided towards professions where they will be independent and self-reliant.

The Impatiens state is clearly distinct from the Vervain state:

Impatiens   Inner tension due to nervous frustration, because things don't move fast enough. Does not impose this on others if left to work undisturbed.

Vervain   Inner tension due to excessive will power. Always inclined to 'inspire' others.

Impatiens Key Symptoms
Impatient, irritable, excessive reactions.

Symptoms Due to Energy Block
- Tension due to rapid mental activity.

- Everything expected to go quickly and smoothly.

- Finds it hard to wait for things to take their course.

- People who work more slowly cause frustration.

- Spontaneous, active, energetic.

- Impatient and lacking in tact with others who are slower.

- Takes the words out of the mouths of others, from impatience.

- Impatiently takes things into own hands.

- Impatience leads to precipitate decisions.

- Telling others to hurry up.

- Prefers to work alone, at own pace.

- Cannot stand fools gladly.

- Great desire for independence.

- Easily flares up and is curt and brusque, though anger passes just as quickly.

- Extreme inner tension makes accident prone, though able to react quickly.

- Short-term exhaustion: sudden hunger because energy resources depleted by fast pace.

- Possible physical reactions such as sudden pain due to nervous tension; nervous indigestion; hot flushes.

- Nervous indigestion.

- Hot flushes.

Potential Following Transformation
- Quick on the uptake, quick thinking and acting.

- Independent mind.

- Above average gifts.

- Patience, delicacy of feeling.

- Gentleness, empathy and understanding for others.

- Able to use one's gifts diplomatically for the benefit of all.

Supportive Measures
- Take a deep breath before saying anything.

- Provide an outlet for frustration with a suitable form of physical exercise.

- Ensure sufficient sleep.

- In resistant cases: consider change of occupation.

Positive Statements for Practice
'I hear with my heart.'

'Depth rather than pace!'

'Each has his own speed.'

19. LARCH,
Larix decidua

A graceful tree reaching a height of up to 30 metres, preferring hills and the edges of woods. Male and female flowers grow on the same tree. They open at the time when the needles just become visible as tiny bright green tufts.

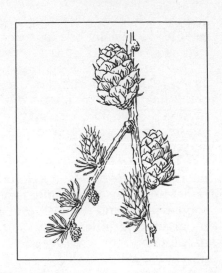

Principle

Larch relates to the soul quality of self-confidence. In the negative Larch state, a person feels inferior to others from the word go.

It is no longer a question of doubting one's abilities, but the feeling is one of absolute conviction of inferiority. One seems to know that one cannot do certain things, and thus doesn't even attempt them. With this, the Larch person is depriving himself of the best thing life has to offer; the chance to learn, to change through new experiences, and to live life to the full. The personality does not unfold, and instead grows impoverished. What remains is a feeling of discouragement and a wholly unconscious melancholy.

The error in this case is that the personality is holding on too much to past negative experiences, rather than letting itself be guided by its Higher Self, trusting in it, in the knowledge that success and failure are of equal value in the end.

Many people have problems in recognizing their own limits. With Larch, exactly the opposite is the case. Specific limits are taken as a matter of course from the beginning, and such limits mean that there can be no development.

Larch types often appear very sensible to those around them, their reasons why they can or will not do certain things seeming very logical: 'Being a woman, I don't really have a chance anyway.' 'I haven't got any A-Levels, like other people.' 'I'd really like to, but I know even now that I shan't manage.'

The foundations of such genuine inferiority feelings have as a rule been laid in infancy and even earlier. Very often the child has taken in its parent's negative attitude with its mother's milk. The certainty of failure has become an inbuilt automatic response, reinforced by each new failure. A vicious circle has been set up.

Just as the larch tree is more delicately structured, so people in frequent need of Larch are also delicately structured psychologically and do not always have the robustness and decisiveness to resist the negative programming inherent in them. That is a pity, for they are usually not only just as capable, but in fact more capable than others.

A typical example is the assistant buyer in a chain-store business who started as a secretary, but as the years progress has shown herself to be more capable and efficient than her boss. When a position as buyer in another department becomes available, her colleagues kindly advise her to apply. Yet she refuses, saying that she has only been trained as a secretary, an argument that is wholly meaningless in relation to her actual qualifications. At the same time she will with a certain unconscious admiration talk about a friend who dared to take a similar step and was successful. There is no envy (Holly) and bitterness (Willow) in her words, but the wrong kind of modesty, quite out of place in her colleagues' opinion, a modesty blanketing her unrealized longing to develop further.

Larch energy helps to dissolve the self-limiting, fixed concepts of the personality and permits the true potential to come to fruition. Somehow one is suddenly able to take a more 'relaxed' view of things and consider alternatives. The initiative can be taken, and the phrase 'I can't' disappears from the vocabulary. Continuing to assess things critically, but from what is basically a positive point of view, it is now possible to cope with almost every situation. A very human attitude develops, with one's own ego held in proper balance.

Larch is used in practice both for long-term treatment and for dealing with temporary problems relating to self-confidence. It has proved useful before examinations, for instance, during divorce proceedings when both partners usually suffer great blows to their self-esteem, and for children who won't venture on their own, but always want to have dad or mum go first.

Some practitioners have also seen good results in the treatment of alcoholics who drink in order to 'forget that they are not as capable as others', and in the treatment of problems with sexual potency with the typical attitude that one is bound to fail again.

Larch Key Symptoms
Expecting to fail, due to lack of self-confidence; inferiority complexes.

Symptoms Due to Energy Block
- Automatically feels inferior to others.

- Admires others, does not believe oneself capable of success.

- Never expects anything but failure.

- Firmly convinced that one cannot do it, therefore does not even try.

- Hesitant and passive, due to lack of self-confidence.

- Illness used as an excuse not to have to tackle something.

- False modesty from lack of self-confidence.

- Feels useless and impotent.

Potential Following Transformation
- Is realistic in tackling things.

- Perseveres, even when there are setbacks.

- Able to assess situations objectively.

Supportive Measures
- Try to understand that we all experience what we have in mind.

- Note that others, too, are only doing their best.

- Look for new experiences, new people, new hobbies, to

get to know more and more facets of your personality.

Positive Statements for Practice
'I am giving up all limiting notions.'

'I can do it. I will do it. I am doing it.'

'Every day is a new beginning.'

20. MIMULUS,
Mimulus guttatus

An immigrant from North America, this perennial, about 30cm in height, grows along brooks, streams and in damp places. The large solitary yellow flowers open between June and August.

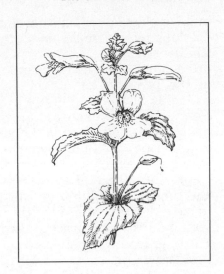

Principle

Mimulus relates to the soul qualities of courage and confidence. In the negative Mimulus state, one has to learn to overcome one's fears.

Mimulus people have one or a number of quite concrete fears, e.g. of going on escalators, or of cancer. These are tangible fears that arise in everyday life, such as being nervous of inviting people to one's house, or fear of an injection at the dentist's. These people would never speak of their fears of their own accord, but if asked a direct question will produce more and more anxieties and fears: fear of being alone, fear of rows over the housekeeping money, fear of snakes etc. The list of Mimulus fears is endless. It includes practically every variety of the theme of the great archetypal fears man is subject to in his life on earth.

Some Bach practitioners think that the Mimulus fears represent a residue of the archetypal fear of the newborn, a fear of the harsh world and of life in the physical body. The Mimulus baby, starting to cry on waking when there is no apparent reason, clearly shows how painful it must be to enter into this physical reality. People who are in the negative Mimulus state sometimes say that life on this earth is like a burden on their backs, and that they often wish they could simply withdraw from it.

People with marked Mimulus traits tend to be of delicate

build or show other external signs of delicacy. Some resemble precious china dolls in human form. Others are like frightened mice, always needing a certain amount of protection. Mimulus types are very sensitive physically, and in the presence of others are apt to blush, stammer or suddenly have a frog in the throat. Others talk far too much from sheer nervousness, giggle nervously, or suffer from damp palms of the hands. There are also others who are good at covering up their negative Mimulus state, appearing strong and extrovert in everyday life. It is only at a second glance that one notices that they really are rather reserved and sensitive, and in their heart of hearts really do not wish to have that much to do with this world. This is a trait often seen in artists such as musicians, actors and painters.

People in the negative Mimulus state apply more subtle standards, and are above all not able to take in as much as others — less blinding lights, less food, fewer activities — one is hypersensitive to many things in the environment when in the Mimulus state, feeling like a humming bird caught up in a colony of rooks.

Many Mimulus people fall ill if the pressure gets too great. They will then develop 'their headache', 'their cystitis', and the like. Mimulus patients are also inclined to be overcareful in convalescence and with this delay the process of recovery.

Mimulus types are usually peaceable, apart from anything else because of their sensitivity, and even if they have an occasional attack of rage this will not be very powerful. They are about as threatening to their environment as an enraged butterfly.

People who often need Mimulus need to learn two things. Firstly, to live with their sensitive constitution, which is indeed something precious. This also means the ability to withdraw from the world at times, without feeling guilty, in order to recharge their batteries and give their nerves a chance to recover. It is very important for them to have a room of their own. Mimulus types also need to come to terms with the phenomenon of fear, and realize that their anxious thoughts are forces that have a tendency to materialize, like all thoughts; any further anxiety will reinforce the first, tying up further energies and getting the person more and more enmeshed in their anxieties.

'In the world you have tribulation; but be of good cheer, I have overcome the world.' These words from John's gospel provide the key to the Mimulus state. As long as the personality uses only worldly standards, it will again and again find itself facing concrete fears. If, however, it allows itself to be guided by the laws of its soul, gives up its worldly limitations and turns more towards the great whole, it will also be able to overcome the world, i.e. its fears.

Taking Mimulus, one will find the way out of the confusion of fears and anxieties, back to one's own true nature. One will find that fear is primarily a problem in one's own mind and can be tackled from the mind, so that one learns to deal with it more effectively. In this way a Mimulus character can grow beyond his anxieties and use his fine sense of humour and his human understanding to help others who are in a similar situation.

When Mimulus comes up in the diagnostic interview, the concrete fear of the moment should be quite specifically mentioned once again in the conversation, and it should be said that Mimulus will now help to resolve this particular anxiety block. If that anxiety then disappears in the course of treatment, experience has shown that several other anxieties will dissolve at the same time.

The distinction of fears seen with Rock Rose, Aspen and Mimulus is as follows:

Rock Rose   Very acute fears bordering on terror.
Aspen   Vague fears of foreboding and apprehension that cannot be clearly defined.
Mimulus   General fears due to known conditions.

Mimulus Key Symptoms
Specific fears that can be named; shyness; timidity; afraid of the world.

Symptoms Due to Energy Block
- Shy, timid, reserved, very sensitive physically.

- The rough and tumble of life is frightening, but fears are kept to oneself.

- Specific anxieties and phobias such as:
  Fear of the cold; fear of the dark; fear of illness and pain; fear of cancer; fear of death; fear of the future; fear of accidents; fear for one's health; fear of losing one's friends; fears of the telephone; fear of spiders; mice, dogs, etc.;

- All kinds of hypersensitivities, such as: to cold; noise; unkindness; loud words; conflict; contradiction; aggression; does not want to be talked to, etc.

- Unsure of oneself due to nervousness, occasional speech difficulties or stammer; nervous laughter.

- Blushes easily.

- Afraid to be alone, but shy and nervous in company.

- Gets very anxious when meeting with opposition or when things are not working out.

- Presence of others is enervating.

- Overcautious during convalescence, e.g. not daring to move the broken leg for fear of hurting it or undoing the healing that has taken place.

- Easily falls ill when faced with the things one is afraid of.

Potential Following Transformation
- Fine character; sensitive.

- Has grown beyond anxieties, able to face the world with cheerful equanimity.

- Personal courage and understanding for others in a similar situation.

Supportive Measures
- Accept that you are different, and that sensitivity is something precious.

- Create free space around you physically, own room to which you can retire to recuperate.

- Mentally come to grips with the phenomenon of anxiety.

- Take care of your kidneys.

Positive Statements for Practice
'Every problem is an opportunity for growth.'

'I am already released from my fear.'

'I feel inner strength and courage.'

'I trust my inner guidance.'

21. MUSTARD,
Sinapis arvensis

An annual 30–60cm in height
growing in fields and by the
wayside. The brilliant yellow
flowers first form short
spikes which soon develop
into long, beaded pods.
Flowers from May to July.

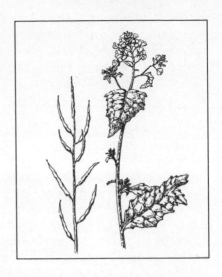

Principle

Mustard relates to the soul qualities of cheerfulness and
serenity. In the negative Mustard state, black depression
descends like a dark cloud.

Out of the blue sky, melancholia descends, an unexpected
gloom. It envelopes a person, putting an isolating layer of
deep despair between them and the rest of the world. One
suddenly feels a stranger in one's own life, with all thoughts
turned back to oneself, and all energies seemingly drained
down an invisible channel. Whilst this dark force surrounds
one, one is completely at its mercy, and there is no way of
getting out of it — neither by diversion nor commonsense
reason. Nor is it possible to cover it over, the way Agrimony
can. The immobile dark weight is too strong, keeping one
imprisoned until it lifts of its own accord, disappearing just as
suddenly as it arrived. There is a sigh of relief and gratitude
— until the next cloud descends.

We have all experienced such unexpected attacks of gloom,
though not always in their extreme form, but the Mustard
state frequently also develops on more inward planes, when
it will not be consciously noted.

This state clearly shows how every negative soul state is a
state of reduced energy frequency, so that all functions are
depressed: physical (with slowness of movement), mental (in
this case lack of drive) and spiritual (with perception

reduced). In the negative Mustard state there is the specific sensation of an unknown outside frequency largely overshadowing those of the personality, for a time almost completely severing the connection with the outside world.

It is therefore not easy to answer the question as to where the error lies in this state. It may be considered from different points of view.

The problem appears to be one not limited to present earth existence. Esoteric thinkers would say that the reasons for the negative Mustard state are karmic, arising from the very depths of the soul. The Mustard state is the consequence of having fallen from a great height. It is the fall of a personality who already had been considerably advanced, but used the above-average faculties that gave it access to cosmic forces in other forms of existence entirely for its own limited ends, squandering them. It has exploited inner resources that should have become nothing but the instrument of the soul and of higher spiritual powers. Considered in this way, the negative Mustard state is one of the soul mourning the lost potential, the personality now having to experience this in painful impotence.

This experience of being immobile, totally separated from the soul, its true source of life, will sooner or later induce the personality to yearn again for the light of its soul and therefore re-approach it. Experience has shown that the Mustard state is immediately lightened once it has been accepted, and the person consciously enters into the mourning state and passes through it.

Seen like this, every negative Mustard state becomes a precious gift, similar to Sweet Chestnut, re-opening the door to the depths of the soul which had been lost sight of.

The Mustard state often occurs before decisive steps are taken in development. In the course of spiritual development, almost everyone goes through negative Mustard phases, so that we may also experience this dark cosmic energy within ourselves, live through it in pain, and transform it.

Some people appear to have a special affinity for this energy quality and be able to transform more of it within themselves than others. It may be a comfort to them to know that every transformation achieved in the individual has an effect on all others and on the great whole. Knowing that with every dark Mustard day lived through they have also brought a little more light to our planet, they will be able to live through their depressive feelings with an inner satisfaction.

Edward Bach wrote: 'This remedy dispels gloom, and brings joy into life.' Anyone taking Mustard has the feeling of slowly waking from a dark, heavy dream.

People who are in the positive Mustard state will have a feeling of inner joyful serenity that is with them through grey days as well as sunny days. They do still see the dark clouds, but do not allow themselves to be depressed by them.

Differentiation between Mustard and Gentian:

Mustard	Gloom that comes and goes for no apparent reason.
Gentian	The reason for the depressive feelings is known, e.g. menopause, midlife crisis, loss of a job, etc.

The essential difference between the Mustard and the Sweet Chestnut states:

Mustard	More passive, more emotional, does not know what is happening, for there are no obvious connections with the rest of one's life.
Sweet Chestnut	More active; able to express one's deep despair in words.

Mustard Key Symptoms
Periods of deep gloom, melancholia, suddenly appear and disappear, for no apparent reason.

Symptoms Due to Energy Block
- Something heavy, black, unknown descends; the soul is in mourning.

- Gloomy depressive feelings come out of a blue sky, enveloping the personality like a black cloud.

- Feels excluded from normal life.

- Can see no logical connection between this condition and the rest of one's life.

- Completely introverted, caught up in gloom, all energies in-turned.

- Unable to cover up this mood before others.

- Unable to overcome the mood with commonsense arguments.

- At the mercy of this feeling until it goes of its own accord; then feels as though set free from prison.

- Afraid of these attacks, because unable to do anything about them.

- Unrecognized anger, at a situation or another person, may be a contributory factor.

Potential Following Transformation
- Inner serenity, cheerfulness and stability on bright and cloudy days.

Supportive Measures
- Acknowledge the mood, enter into it fully, e.g. by listening to sad music, drive to the beach on a rainy day, etc.

- Yearn for your soul like a lover.

Positive Statements for Practice
'I feel full of joy.'

'I am rising into the light.'

'My heart feels light and happy.'

'I am grateful for the hours of pain.'

22. OAK,
Quercus robur

The oak was considered a holy tree by our forefathers. It grows in woodlands and grassland. Male and female flowers develop on the same tree, flowering between the end of April and early May.

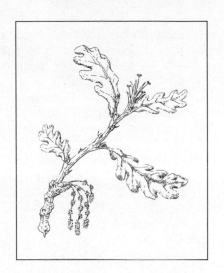

Principle

Oak relates to the soul potential of strength and endurance. In the negative Oak state these character traits are handled too rigidly.

Instead of allowing itself to be taken by the hand, figuratively speaking, by its Higher Self and letting itself be guided through difficult and enjoyable periods in life, the personality mistakenly gets itself stuck in a self-chosen permanent high achievement stress. Life is a constant struggle, and the oak person has all the attributes of the winner: inborn powers of resistance, almost superhuman endurance,* tremendous will power, courage, devotion to duty, unbroken hope and high ideals.

The Oak personality has forgotten that it is not only achievement and winning that makes life worth living, and that redoubtable fighters, too, will find strength for new deeds from the more subtle, playful, or tender-hearted moments in life.

If he does not allow himself those creative interludes, his inner life will grow more and more spartan and impoverished. He will be working, but his heart won't be in it. Endurance imperceptibly becomes an aim in itself and the

---

*It is interesting to note that oak trees are so highly resistant that they are able to survive in places where earth radiations are so powerful that other trees, such as beeches, will die.

person a rigid high performance engine, automatically running on until normal wear and tear bring it to a stop. Then there will be a sudden attack, a nervous collapse, mental 'piston seizure', and if there is even greater will power, this may show itself in form of physical symptoms based on rigidity and loss of flexibility.

People needing Oak often are of strong and gnarled appearance. 'He is the mainstay of the firm, a real worker, and the only one you really can rely on,' others will admiringly say of a person with marked Oak traits. 'No good complaining. It's got to be done!' an Oak person will say, rolling up his sleeves and getting on with it. Oak people will catch up on their A-Levels in evening classes, even if it takes them years. Oak mothers are unceasingly active looking after the family. They may not have had a holiday for years, but would never admit to being overworked.

People with Oak characteristics do not take the easy way out. It is they who will keep the whole family going through difficult times or sustain a whole nation. Their enormous contribution is not always properly recognized and suitably recompensed, and that is in part their own fault. The strong Oak type feels an inner reluctance ever to appear weak in the eyes of others. Being worried, not always justifiably, of becoming dependent, he'd do anything rather than ask others for help.

Oak characters are noble, indeed regally, minded. They help others of their own accord, and nothing will make them more discontented and unhappy than to be unable to meet the obligations they have accepted due to impaired health. Nothing will make them more depressed than having to disappoint others in what they believe they expect. It is such a joy to them to feel the pleasure they have given to those around them reflected back onto themselves; pleasure they believe they have to deny themselves on their strenuous, stony path through life.

We may ask what makes people opt for such tremendous achievement, never losing courage in the face of adversity, the way most of us do. From the esoteric point of view, this may be answered as follows: Oak types are convinced in their heart of hearts of the greatness and immortality of their soul, and consider it their duty to cherish this heritage. The present life is often experienced as a 'temporary fall from grace', with that inner certainty of the immortality of the soul providing the strength to survive the life on earth. The external vicissitudes of this journey through life are designed to break down the fixed behaviour patterns that have developed over many lives, and make the soul flexible and capable of growing again.

As soon as the personality consciously or unconsciously recognizes this and, instead of mindlessly battling on, becomes flexible in following the inner inpulses of its Higher Self, the journey through life will become both easier and more pleasant.

Taking Oak, one soon finds the inner pressure reducing, with energies flowing more abundantly and in a way more freely. Heart, soul and vitality are given new life. The playful element returns, and with it pleasure in life. It will then be possible to meet one's commitments without putting so much effort into them. One is indeed as strong as an oak, with new primal forces constantly arising from the very soil.

Oak has proved a useful help during recovery from long-term illness, when the patient, though resolutely persisting in good will, slowly grows tired of continued treatments such as physical therapy, baths, etc. Oak will provide new momentum and power to persevere.

Oak is sometimes confused with Elm. The key difference is:
Elm   Work is taken as a vocation. The state of exhaustion is temporary.
Oak   Work is often seen as a duty, a commitment. The exhaustion may be chronic.

The absolute opposite of Oak is Gorse. Here, one gives up in face of difficulties. Oak never gives up.

Oak Key Symptoms
The fighter, exhausted and brought to his knees, who nevertheless struggles on bravely, never giving up.

Symptoms Due to Energy Block
- Dutiful, reliable.

- A plodder.

- Tends to overwork and is then depressed and despondent.

- Is utterly worn out and exhausted, but never complains.

- Almost superhuman endurance and patience.
- Untiring and persistent in endeavours, never giving up.
- Fights bravely against all odds, never losing hope.
- Often only continues to work from a sense of duty.
- Helps to shoulder the burdens of others.
- Is dissatisfied when health problems prevent obligations being met, or limit ability to help.
- Ignores natural impulse to rest.
- Endeavours not to let tiredness and weakness show on the outside.

Potential Following Transformation
- Endurance, reliability, steadfastness, strength, commonsense.
- Able to stand great stress exceedingly well.
- Overcomes all life's vicissitudes with courage and persistence.

Supportive Measures
- Oak people should be encouraged not to be quite so dogged in their approach to life and sometimes just do what they fancy. Take a break, loaf about, take up silly hobbies, etc.
- Exercises for tensed neck and shoulder region.

Positive Statements for Practice
'Joy will yield strength.'

'I shall do it.'

'Energy is flowing to me from the primal source.'

23. OLIVE,
Olea europoea

The olive tree, an evergreen
native to the Mediterranean,
flowers in different spring
months according to the
climate of the country where
the tree grows. The
inflorescence consists of 20
or 30 inconspicuous white
flowers.

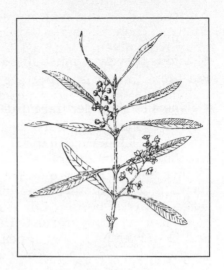

Principle
The dove brought Noah an olive branch to indicate that the
Flood was over, and peace and quiet had returned to the
earth. In the similar way, the Flower Remedy Olive relates to
the principle of regeneration, peace and restored balance.

This is the 'calm following the storm', when body, mind
and spirit are utterly exhausted and spent after a long period
of great strain — after physical illness, a long period on an
unbalanced diet, after severe lack of sleep, and also after
devoted care given to nursing a member of the family, after
years of voluntary work done on top of a full-time job, and
after powerful inner development processes that
unconsciously have used up a great deal of energy.

The negative Olive state always represents a 'last straw'
reaction. You don't want to see any more or hear any more,
but just go to sleep, or be allowed to sit there. The smallest
job, even the daily washing up, becomes an insurmountable
obstacle. 'I am so exhausted, I could cry.' 'I am completely
finished', 'I feel sick I'm so tired.' Those are typical phrases
expressing the negative Olive state.

People who quite often find themselves in this state will
have to learn to husband their vital energies properly. Their
mistake is that they completely spend themselves at the
personality level, where energies are limited, rather than
draw strength from higher sources. It is during periods of

particular strain that man should call for energy from higher sources. There is enough energy available in the universe, and we can obtain it if we ask for it in the right frame of mind, knowing that we cannot exist on our own resources alone. At the same time it is important to recognize and accept the individual laws and workings of our own body.

The Olive state is always a call to humility, and at the same time a challenge to learn to deal properly with our vital energy, which is after all the divine energy. Olive people find this difficult, for the physical warning system used by the Higher Self to signal that we are overdoing it physically, mentally or spiritually, is no longer functioning very well.

People in the positive Olive state find that it is possible to cope with even the greatest stress in the fullness of strength and even with joy. They appear to others to have seemingly inexhaustible resources. They are able to take heed of early warning signals and are flexible in adapting to the energy requirements made of them. They completely give themselves up to inner guidance, knowing that the necessary energies will come to them from the universe when the right moment is there.

In practice, it is also essential to pay particular attention to the physical condition of a person in a negative Olive state. Poor physical function also often serves to indicate that the flow of energy is disturbed throughout the whole system, taking the form, for instance, of abnormal oxygen levels in the blood, reduced kidney function, a toxic intestinal flora etc. If it has not already been done, a medical check-up is called for with the Olive state. Conversely, Olive always gives great assistance in debilitating physical conditions, strengthening body and soul. In the experience of some practitioners, Olive has also proved extremely useful in treating the recovery stage of alcoholism.

The distinction between Olive and Hornbeam:

Olive   For total exhaustion of body, mind and spirit.
Hornbeam   Tiredness is more in the mind. In the morning one feels one won't be able to manage. In the course of the day it is found that one is managing after all.

Olive Key Symptoms

Completely exhausted, extreme physical and mental fatigue.

Symptoms Due to Energy Block
- Exhaustion following long period of strain or physical illness.

- Feels completely washed out, finished.

- No reserves left.

- Everything is an effort.

- Deep inner tiredness after periods of great inner struggle and transformation that used up many psychic energies.

- Exhaustion after long period of devoted nursing care.

- Needs much sleep.

Potential Following Transformation
- Great strength and vitality.

- During periods of stress, relies completely on inner guidance, and is thus able to cope even with extreme demands with cheerfulness.

Supportive Measures
- Consider the subject of energy, Prana, etc.

- Yoga exercises to replenish the energy system.

- Get plenty of sleep.

- Relaxation in the open air.

- Food rich in etheric energies: grains, vegetables, fruit.

Positive Statements for Practice
'I ask for strength to do what I have to do.'

'I feel cosmic energy flowing into me.'

'I recognize the needs of my body.'

24. PINE,
Pinus sylvestris

A slender tree reaching a
height of up to 30 metres, its
bark brown-red lower down
and orange-brown in the
upper crown. Grows in
forests and on heaths, liking
a sandy soil. The male and
female flowers grow on the
same tree; the male is thickly
covered with yellow pollen.

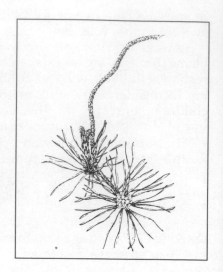

Principle

Pine relates to the soul qualities of regret and forgiveness. A
person in the negative Pine state will cling to his guilt
feelings.

The feeling of guilt may be of recent origin, perhaps
because one forgot to close the window and the budgerigar
escaped. Or the guilt feelings may be archetypal, going back
a long way, even to original sin or Eve's guilt in offering the
apple to Adam. Pine, together with Holly, is probably one of
the most existential human soul states, and is not always
easily recognized in another.

An unconscious Pine state often betrays itself in
unconscious guilt-tinged phrases such as: 'I'll never forgive
myself for having been so careless', or: 'Excuse me if I take
this seat'; 'I know it is my fault that the boy makes such a
noise ...'; 'Well, my parents actually wanted a girl, but they
had to make do with a son.'

Guilt often tempers the Pine-type person's whole feeling
for life, with the result that physically he tends to be tired and
worn out. The joy of living plays practically no role in the life
of Pine people. They are the type of people who are never
really satisfied with themselves, despite many positive
experiences, and blame themselves for not having taken
more trouble. A person in the negative Pine state asks more
of himself than of others, and if the high standards applied to

himself cannot be lived up to, he will desperately blame himself in his heart.

Another characteristic trait of the Pine state is to take the blame for the mistakes of others, feeling that one shares responsibility. He will feel guilty, for instance, if he has to ask his inconsiderate neighbour to turn down the stereo. Pine children tend to be the scapegoat in class, and will uncomplainingly take punishments for crimes they have not even committed. When Pine types are ill or overworked they will apologize to everybody. If there are only four loaves of bread for five people the Pine person will stand back, for he would feel guilty in his heart if another person had to go without.

It seems that a person in the negative Pine state is always apologizing, even for existing, perhaps lacking conviction in his heart of hearts that he deserves to be on this earth. One can often sense a childish nervousness unconsciously characterized by dogmatic, excessively moral mental concepts and powerful commandments: 'You have to work.' 'You should not desire sex.' 'God sees everything and also knows that you have long since failed as a human being.' That being so, one really deserves nothing but punishment and penitence, painful and severe, an eye for an eye, a tooth for a tooth.

And when there is no punishment from above, one punishes oneself. This is the reason why many people in the negative Pine state unconsciously make a cross for their own back. Sometimes they also say they are taking on the karma of others. Some Pine types have an almost masochistic desire to sacrifice themselves and may punish themselves for life by choosing an inconsiderate partner, not being aware of the inner reason for this. They will offer love, or what they take to be love, without being able to accept love for themselves. A tragic and life-destroying error of the personality in several respects:

If the personality shuts itself off from love, from the stream of life, divine energies cannot flow through it. It therefore not only cuts off its own vital nerve, but also commits a sin against unity, against the whole of creation. Its self-destructive guilt programmes irritate and damage everybody around them.

The reason for such an attitude again lies in the personality completely taking the wrong view, limiting itself to live by its own concept of good and evil, claiming the right to judge for itself, rather than accept what it learns under the guidance of its Higher Self.

A person in the negative Pine state has to realize what it means, in the profoundest sense, to be a human being, and that the very fact that we live and breathe on this earth makes any doubt as to our right to exist an utter absurdity. We need to accept that whilst man has a perfect soul, he is in his physical body an imperfect creature, and that no progress can be made in this body without setbacks and failures. It is the very conflicts over our errors that provide us with the necessary energies for further development. We therefore need to make mistakes, and will continue to make new mistakes all the time, and these mistakes will finally bring us closer and closer to our own soul and therefore to God.

Why then accuse oneself? Anyone holding on to their mistakes, unable to love and forgive themselves, will also be unable to love and forgive others. What, then, would be the point of a human relationship?

Pine can help us to grasp the true content of the Christian concept of salvation. We can accept that a person need not carry guilt, for his guilt has been forgiven even before he came into this world, by the symbolic sacrifice on the cross. All he needs to do is to acknowledge this.

In the positive Pine state one is aware that the age of the vengeful God seen by Moses and of his strict commandments has passed, that there is no more need for punishment, for each of us can come closer to salvation to the extent to which we are able to feel genuine, pure regret.

People who have been able to transform a severe negative Pine state receive a great deal of energy. They are able to help others with similar problems, by patiently listening to them, sharing experience, and indeed often just by their energetic radiation, merely by being there.

In practice, Pine is often followed by Willow or Holly. The distinction between the Crab Apple feeling of being unclean and the Pine feeling of guilt is as follows:

Pine   Clings onto his guilt feelings as though they are a part of him.

Crab Apple   Feels unclean, dirty, but does not accept responsibility for this condition. Would like to get rid of it as fast as possible.

Pine Key Symptoms
Self-reproach, guilt feelings, despondency.

Symptoms Due to Energy Block
- Often uses apologetic turns of phrase in conversation.
- Often feels guilty, tends to blame oneself.
- Introverted, little joy in life.
- Feels partly responsible for the mistakes of others.
- Sets the highest standards for oneself — more than for others — and feels guilty at heart if unable to live up to them.
- Even if successful, feels one could have done this or that even better.
- Looks more to one's limits than one's potentials; self-destructively undermines oneself with negative self-image.
- Feels unworthy, inferior, an underdog waiting for the stick.
- Excuses oneself for being ill, depressed or exhausted.
- At heart of hearts considers oneself a coward.
- Finds it difficult to accept anything, unconsciously feeling one does not deserve anything.
- Feels guilty when need arises to speak firmly to others.
- Feels one does not deserve love, refusing oneself the right to exist: 'Forgive me for having been born.'
- Sometimes masochistic desire to sacrifice.
- Extremely undervalues oneself, negative narcissism.
- Commonly has unconscious concepts of good and evil with strongly religious flavour to them, sees sexuality as sin, notions of original sin, etc.

Potential Following Transformation
- Admits own faults, accepting them, but does not cling to them.

- Feels genuine regret rather than guilt; able to forgive oneself and forget.

- Deep understanding of human nature, particularly human feelings.

- Shares the burdens of others, but only if this is meaningful.

- Great patience, humility, simplicity of heart.

- True understanding of the Christian concept of salvation.

Supportive Measures
- Give recognition to yourself, knowing that every human being merits love and 'that your sin has already been forgiven'.

- Yoga exercises to reinforce the flow of energy between the 'third eye', thyroid and heart chakras.

- Establish where you are asking too much of yourself, setting unattainable goals. Give up those goals, formulate new goals.

- Fitness training in the mornings, to build up reserve vitality for the day.

Positive Statements for Practice.
'I love myself just as I am.'

'I forgive myself, for I have long since been forgiven.'

'I have been born and already redeemed.'

'Every error is a step nearer to God.'

25. RED CHESTNUT,
Aesculus carnea

More delicate and less robust than the white horse chestnut. The flowers are a good strong rose pink, appearing in large pyramidal inflorescences in late May or early June.

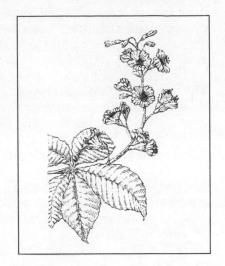

Principle
Red Chestnut relates to the soul potentials of solicitude and love of one's neighbour. A typical feature of the Red Chestnut state is a powerful energy link between two individuals.

People who frequently need Red Chestnut find it easy to tune into other people and situations, and are able to project strongly. From the energy point of view they are great transmitters. People for whom they feel concerned, relatives, children, friends, know all about it.

Red Chestnut characters are seemingly altruistic in their care for others, always thinking the worst will befall them. These are the fathers who can't go to sleep at night until their teenage daughters are back safe and sound from a visit to the cinema. These are the mothers who won't be at peace until their grown-up children have called, late at night, to report that they have safely reached their holiday destination. These are the grandmothers whose heart stops in their mouth when they think that their grandson has to cross a busy road on his own.

Red Chestnut characters suffer for those they love, and think the others won't notice. They forget that they are doing harm not only to themselves, but also to the objects of their care. There is indeed a risk of actually attracting the things they are dreading for others with their energies. Bach told how the worries of his friends made themselves felt as acute physical pain for him when he was involved in an accident.

The Red Chestnut state could also be described as a symbiotic relationship similar to that between mother and infant. The infant wholly depends on its mother for survival. The mother, too, is emotionally living through the child. This close bond tends to persist for too long, however, in many cases, with the cord not cut, or insufficiently cut.

The particular disadvantage for both parties is that their development will be retarded, as a symbiotic state needs to be maintained in equilibrium if it is to function. When one partner attempts to sever the cord, the other will automatically be involved.

A case history of a divorced mother and her depressive 16-year-old son shows that, in the course of treatment, the mother had realized that she was using her son to meet her own emotional needs. Her son, being unconsciously aware of this, had withdrawn more and more from her and from reality, into his own fantasy world.

She took Red Chestnut. A few days later her son grew extremely depressed. After this, however, he was prepared for the first time to undergo treatment, something he had refused to do for years. Red Chestnut had enabled the mother to loosen the bond between them, and at that moment the son, too, was for the first time able to consider his own needs.

Similar symbiotic bonds are also common between married couples, particularly when powerful parent projections are involved, i.e. the wife projects her own father problems onto the husband. An unrecognized symbiotic bond may also exist between a child and one of his parents who is no longer alive.

Fundamentally speaking, the Red Chestnut state is nothing but a 'connection at the wrong level', at a subjective, emotional, anxiety-ridden personality level, rather than at a spiritual level, between the Higher Selves of two people. In the negative Red Chestnut state, the concept of love of your neighbour is egotistically misread. The other person is unconsciously made the object onto which one's own limiting thoughts and doubts are projected.

Here it has to be realized that things 'always work out differently from what you think', and that it is impossible, however great the effort made, to stop others from meeting their destined fate.

'The best laid plans ... I hope he or she does well. Let's hope the best for them. They'll find the right way.'

Anyone thinking like this will experience the positive side of Red Chestnut energy, and will have the pleasure of seeing things go better and better for himself and the other person.

A number of practitioners have reported that Red Chestnut is often used for people who need to identify strongly with others for professional reasons, e.g. nurses or educational counsellors.

Red Chestnut has also proved helpful during weaning. It may be combined with White Chestnut when worries concerning the other person keep coming back and no effort will make them go away.

As a rule, the Red Chestnut state is only temporary. There are few out-and-out Red Chestnut types.

Comparison between Red Chestnut and Chicory in the aspect of over-caring for others:

Red Chestnut	Selfless in their concern, worrying only over dangers that might befall their loved ones.
Chicory	Selfish and possessive in their concern for their loved ones.

Red Chestnut Key Symptoms
- Excessive concern and worry over others.

Symptoms Due to Energy Block
- Great attachment to people, especially those held dear.

- Excessive concern for the safety of others (children, partner), with no fear for own person.

- Worries over the problems of others.

- Over-protective, overcaring.

- Self-sacrificing.

- Thinks something may have happened to the other person if they are late.

- Afraid a harmless symptom may be a sign of serious illness in another.

- Realizing that it has been a matter of 'saved by the skin of his teeth', one imagines all the terrible things that might have happened to the other person.

- Parents constantly warning their children to be careful.

Potential Following Transformation
- Ability to radiate positive thoughts of security, well-being and courage to others when in difficult situations.

- Able to provide a positive influence and guidance for others from a distance.

- Keeps a cool head in emergencies; able to cope mentally and physically.

Supportive Measures
- Reflect on 'the power of thought', on spiritual healing; do exercises to train awareness, etc.

- Train yourself to bring to mind the positive side of the coin when negative thoughts come up. Thus, do not imagine the worst that may happen (car accident), but visualize the desirable end (safe return).

- Imagine the person you feel concern for surrounded by white light.

Positive Statements for Practice
'He or she is in God's hands.'

'I am radiating peace, calm and optimism.'

'Everything is taking a positive turn.'

'I am a unique personality.'

26. ROCK ROSE,
Helianthemum nummularium

Freely branching under-
shrub growing on chalky
downs, limestone and
gravelly soils. The radiant
yellow flowers open from
June to September, usually
only one or two at a time.

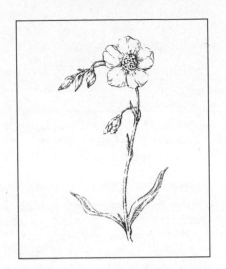

Principle

Rock Rose relates to the soul qualities of courage and
steadfastness. It is one of the most important components of
Rescue Remedy.

A personality in the negative Rock Rose state is under acute
threat, mentally and often physically also. These are
moments of crisis, exceptional situations like accidents,
sudden illness, natural disasters, when the human being is
unable to cope with the onrush of elemental energies.
Everything is happening too fast, going in the wrong
direction. Worlds are separating the personality from its
Higher Self as it fearfully cowers within its mortal confines
instead of trusting in the guidance of its soul which could let
flow towards it the energies which are needed to master the
situation.

A refugee escapes over the border. The ground has been
mined. Search lights are sweeping the area at regular
intervals. Suddenly, the sound of barking dogs is coming
from behind. Has he been spotted? His heart is in his mouth.
In total panic, and feeling utterly the hunted creature, he
runs and runs for his life ...

That is an extreme example of the Rock Rose state. All Rock
Rose states are as dramatic as that inside, even if external
circumstances are not quite as threatening. In every case, the
personality is in an acute emergency state. At the physical

level, these are the situations where one dials the medical emergency service. The 'victim' will often be out of his mind with panic, his vision, hearing and speech below normal. A sudden life-threatening illness in the family, when the worst is feared, calls for Rock Rose — for the family as well as the patient.

Children waking screaming from a nightmare should be given sips of Rock Rose until they have calmed down again. Someone who has escaped a car accident by a hair's breadth and still feels the fear in his bones, is in the negative Rock Rose state.

The state has been aptly described as 'a punch in the stomach', for the solar plexus function has been overstrained. Too much is coming in too quickly, and the central nervous system is unable to cope. Sensitives say that the solar plexus chakra 'freezes in a position that is wide open'. Some then experience the solar plexus as a 'sore hole', or a 'stone in the pit of the stomach'.

A person in the Rock Rose state feels himself helplessly in the power of the elements. They are sweating blood for fear. The fear-emanation pervades the whole aura, and many sensitives have given vivid descriptions of this.

Rock Rose energy liberates the personality from its state of frozen fear, letting the pendulum swing back from the negative to the positive state.* Self-centered fear becomes courage, even heroic courage, in the extreme case forgetting self for the sake of others.

This is the courage that will make a mother stop a car with her bare hands when it threatens to run over her child who is happily at play. It is the heroism that will make partisans stand up against an enemy army of overwhelming power, and win. Rock Rose is able to mobilize tremendous forces that allow men to grow beyond themselves.

By nature the Rock Rose state occurs only temporarily. It is quite often indicated for children, for they are less stable as yet in their psyche. But there are also genuine Rock Rose types among adults, though they may not always appear all that nervous on the outside. They often are very delicate in

---

*It is interesting to note that the flowers of the common rock rose are a particular radiant yellow. Yellow is the colour capable of storing the maximum amount of heat radiation from the sun in flowers.

their nervous constitution, and sometimes have been born with somewhat underdeveloped adrenal glands. They use up the defensive powers of their mind at an above average rate, their nervous energy resources being easily exhausted.

Rock Rose states may develop when one is undergoing spiritual disciplines, and suddenly finds oneself confronted with a great amount of archetypal darkness.

Sometimes Rock Rose is recommended as additional medication in the conventional treatment of sun and heat stroke. Often it has proved helpful for people given to drugs.

Rock Rose Key Symptoms
Extremely acute state of fear, terror and panic.

Symptoms Due to Energy Block
- Suddenly escalating anxieties in physical or mental emergency situations.

- Terror, horror, naked fear.

- Rigid for fear, terror and panic stricken.

- As though out of his senses for fear — does not hear, does not see, does not speak.

- Heart nearly stops for fear.

- Nervous energy reserves poor.

- Fear still in one's bones after escaping by the skin of one's teeth.

- Panic due to nightmares (especially children).

- Often needed for people given to drugs.

Potential Following Transformation
- Heroism.

- Able to grow beyond oneself in emergencies and crisis situations, and to mobilize almost superhuman powers.

- Does things for the benefit of others, regardless of possible risks to one's own person.

Supportive Measures
As a rule not possible in the acute state.

- People who often need Rock Rose should learn to protect their solar plexus mentally, e.g. by visualizing a 'shield of light' covering the solar plexus.

- Breathing therapy.

- Prayer, mantras.

Positive Statements for Practice
'I am more than my body.'

'I am in God's hands.'

'Undreamt-of forces are streaming towards me.'

27. ROCK WATER

This is not a plant, but water from natural springs located in areas untouched by civilization and known for its power to heal the sick. Such half-forgotten wells, exposed only to the free interplay of sun and wind as they bubble up among trees and grasses, may still be found in many parts of England.

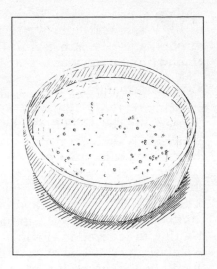

Principle

Rock Water relates to the soul qualities of adaptability and inner freedom. A person in the negative Rock Water state is caught up in rigid, theoretical maxims and ideas divorced from reality.

Such people have erected a 'stone monument' of high spiritual ideals, moral guidelines and perfectionist health concepts, and then feel puny in the face of this monumental image.

A person in the negative Rock Water state will deny himself many of the things that make everyday life pleasant and enjoyable, in the belief that they do not fit in with their strict, often downright ascetic vision of life. Being a non-drinker at a wedding, he will be the only one not raising his glass of champagne to toast the happy couple, smiling modestly as he asks for a glass of mineral water.

Rock Rose types want to be in top form both mentally and physically, and will keenly pursue any course that might lead them there. The man appearing in the swimming pool at 7 a.m., having jogged through the woods, who doggedly swims his fifty lengths, and who thereafter sits down intently to a specially prepared breakfast — that is a classical Rock Water type.

A person in the extreme Rock Water state also wants to be an example to others; they quietly hope to induce others to take up their own ideas so that they, too, shall find 'the right path'. Western members of Eastern religious sects, walking through the city streets in ethnic garb and silent dignity, embody this particular aspect of the Rock Water state.

Many Rock Water types want to be saints whilst still on earth. They will set themselves high principled standards, particularly those that are somehow tangible and can be crossed off. They will for instance spend hours a day in yoga exercises, strictly adhere to macrobiotic principles, or go through specific ritual prayers wherever they may be.

Their high-flown theories and ideas often have the characteristic that they derive from ancient traditions that achieved great things in their day and place but are no longer compatible with the twentieth century and therefore difficult to bring to realization. People who are in the negative Rock Water state will, however, fail to perceive this and torture themselves with self-reproaches when the demands of humdrum everyday life have made it impossible to meet their daily training quota. This of course will do more harm to their development than hours of breathing, praying, meditating etc. are able to offset.

A person in the Rock Water state does not make a good partner in discussions. Whether the issue is politics, environmental pollution or a more philosophical theme, a 'very dogged' view is taken of what he has found to be the right thing for himself. Certain things that do not fit into his own scheme are simply ignored.

Yet unlike Vine he would not attempt to impose his own philosophy on the other person, being far too busy trying to meet his exaggerated self-imposed standards. There is more of a tendency in the negative Rock Water state towards conceitedness, a sublime form of spiritual pride, a self-righteousness.

A person in the Rock Water state does not realize the inner coercion constantly applied, and the fact that he is constantly suppressing important human needs. He fails to note the extent to which he is daily using force on himself, nor the degree to which pleasure in life is suffocated under self-imposed disciplines. These constant exaggerated demands on himself will sooner or later come to expression in many different forms of inflexibility at a physical level.

A person in the negative Rock Water state is strongly

identified in his mind with superpersonal principles, on the mental plane. Highly crystallized, the personality freezes in certain decisions, passing by the demands of reality. It absolutely wants to be what it considers to be good, and in no way what it has identified as not good. Yet it may be exactly the things it believes to be not good that are still necessary for its development. And it is possible that the things it considers good are not yet destined to come up in the present life cycle.

The error lies in excessive self-willedness and a totally wrong material approach. The personality wants to enforce spiritual development, egotistically, confusing external effect with inner cause. It fails to see that an outer effect, e.g. a change in lifestyle, will come of its own accord once the inner conditions for this are given. It has forgotten that certain forms of life are the consequence, not the cause, of spiritual growth.

In wanting to enforce external changes that are against the soul's inner design, the personality is fighting its Higher Self rather than letting itself be guided by it. It is above all failing to understand that 'self-mastery' is achieved not by concentrating on oneself, but by forgetting self in the service of others.

People who are in the negative Rock Water stage need to be encouraged to look their true personality in the face at last, in the spirit of 'nobody is perfect', and forego high-minded theories, instead entrusting themselves to the waves of real life which will wash away the rough edges of every rock.

Those in need of Rock Water should cast off their iron restraints once and for all and no longer deny themselves the pleasures of life. Interestingly, a sensitive taking Rock Water felt 'gently caressed all over his body', experiencing a 'rebirth into reality' as he put it.

People in the positive Rock Water state may be described as adaptable idealists. They are able to put aside their principles and much-lauded convictions when confronted with new insights and greater truths. They keep an open mind. They use discipline in constantly monitoring their ideals in their real-life situation. In this way they will be able, in the course of time, to truly bring many of their ideals to proper realization, and this will of its own accord make them an example to others.

Extreme Rock Water cases of the type described above are

not very common. Yet Rock Water is quite frequently indicated, for we all have areas of our personality where needs are consciously or unconsciously suppressed.

Rock Water Key Symptoms
For those who are hard on themselves, strict, rigid views, suppressed inner needs.

Symptoms Due to Energy Block
• Great perfectionist.

• Life is made subject to dogmatic theories and sometimes exaggerated ideals.

• Denies oneself a great deal, in the belief that it is not compatible with one's concept of life; much of the pleasure in life is lost.

• Hard with oneself; does everything possible to achieve top form and stay in it; self-discipline is writ large.

• Has set the highest standards for oneself and is forcing oneself, almost to the point of self-abandonment, to live according to them.

• Unaware of the compulsions one is living under.

• Wrong concept of spirituality: clings to a particular aspect that is accessible (meditating technique, special diet, etc.) and makes it into a holy cow.

• Believes that worldly desires inhibit spiritual development, wants to be a saint while still on this earth.

• Suppresses important physical and emotional needs, self denying.

• Falls into his own trap when meditating, because of 'wanting' too much.

• Does not interfere in the lives of others, being completely preoccupied with personal perfection.

• Reproaches oneself if unable to maintain self-imposed discipline.

• Physical needs are not well integrated; often dysmenorrhoic.

- Much stress in the physical body — especially in muscles and joints.

Potential Following Transformation
- Open-minded idealist; able to let go of theories and principles if confronted with new insights or deeper truths.

- Does not allow oneself to be influenced by others, knowing that the right insights are to be found within oneself, at the right time.

- Able to bring great ideals to fruition.

- Joy in life and inner peace make one a natural example for others.

Supportive Measures
- In every respect, don't cling.

- Allow yourself more worldly pleasures and enjoyments.

- Practice making clearer distinction between theory and practice; do not subscribe too wholeheartedly to the theories of others, but judge for yourself what is good and what is not.

- Physical exercise not imposing rigid rules.

Positive Statements for Practice
'I am open to new insights and experiences.'

'I let all aspects of my life have their due.'

'I let things grow.'

28. SCLERANTHUS,
Scleranthus annuus

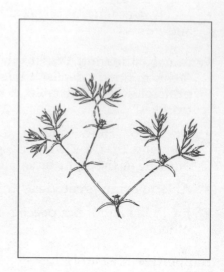

A low annual, bushy or creeping, reaching a height of 5 to 70cm with numerous tangled stems, grows in wheat fields, on sandy and gravelly soils. The flowers appear in clusters, pale to dark green between July and September.

Principle

Scleranthus relates to the soul potentials of poise and balance. A person in the negative Scleranthus state vacillates between two extremes.

Anyone who has watched a grasshopper respond to the slightest movement in the vicinity by making huge leaps hither and thither with apparent aimlessness, can imagine what it feels like inside to be in the negative Scleranthus state. Any outside impulse will be enough to get a reaction, first this way, and then the next.

The new neighbours are charming, you immediately are on the friendliest terms with them, but the next day they get on your nerves to such an extent you'd really like to slam the door in their face.

The night before, you firmly agreed to join your friends in buying a holiday cottage. When you wake up in the morning you wonder what had got into you and try to get out of it all on the telephone. But, in the course of the telephone conversation, you allow yourself to be persuaded again saying you'll reconsider the question. There will be further to-ing and fro-ing, until your friends finally find someone else more able to make up their mind.

A person in the negative Scleranthus state is like a balance that is constantly in motion, swinging from one extreme to the other — in seventh heaven or miserable as hell, extremely active or completely apathetic; one day enthusiastic over a new idea, the next completely disinterested. This constant change of moods and opinions makes Scleranthus types appear unstable and unreliable in the eyes of others.

The girl unable to decide between two men is a classic Scleranthus case. When she is with the quiet civil servant it is perfectly obvious to her that she will be well looked after with him. When she goes out with the adventurous engineer who wants to emigrate with her, she wonders what is really keeping her at home. When she is on her own and tries to consider what she really wants, she'll never come to a decision, but keep ineffectively swinging to and fro between the two possibilities, for weeks, indeed for months. She does not even share her doubts with her parents or with good friends, for, unlike Cerato, Scleranthus will always try to find her own solution, however long that may take.

Dr Philip Chancellor in his *Handbook of the Bach Flower Remedies* describes the case of a man who had taken three months to make up his mind to come for treatment.

The vacillating nature of Scleranthus types also tends to find outward expression in many nervous, dithery gestures. A great many superfluous movements are made. Many women in need of Scleranthus change their clothes several times a day, reacting to their fluctuating moods. A Scleranthus child will often be fidgeting.

Patients of the Scleranthus type are irritating to their doctors, because their symptoms move around all over the body. 'And where does it hurt today?' the therapist will ask, wondering if it is even worthwhile taking the new symptoms seriously.

The lack of balance in the Scleranthus state sometimes finds expression in such physical disequilibrium as travel sickness or complaints of the inner ear. The variable moods are also reflected in variation between physical extremes, e.g. constipation and diarrhoea, above normal and subnormal temperatures, ravenous hunger and loss of appetite. This is also the reason why Scleranthus is frequently indicated during pregnancy.

Some practitioners are of the opinion that a disposition for the negative Scleranthus state may develop during the first two or three hours of life, when the environment is chaotic and too many impressions come in at once. The personality is like a faulty lens that can no longer focus light, i.e. order thoughts and impulses, gather them in a focal point and condense them into a purposeful and unambiguous decision. Its energy is aimlessly and sometimes bizarrely meandering around among different facets of consciousness.

In the Scleranthus state, the error lies in the personality refusing to give clear assent to the guiding role of its Higher Self. As a result, it has no inner line on the goals of its soul, a line that would give it strength, standards and direction. For as long as it has not made a clear decision with regard to the path of its soul, it will fall under the influence of many different forces, becoming the plaything of earthly dualities, attracted now to the one pole now to the other. It therefore squanders valuable time and resources, treading water where its development is concerned.

A person in the negative Scleranthus state has to do everything possible to reach his own centre, in his mind and also physically, and find his true inner rhythm. The first step would be no longer to enter quite so deeply into all the extremes of his positive and negative experiences, but try to establish a golden mean. The attitude should be that of a tightrope walker who first of all sensitively attunes himself to the rhythm of his own movements and then — feet firmly on the rope, eyes firmly focused ahead — lightly moves towards his goal.

This lightness, the outcome of great inner strength, is often typical of people in the positive Scleranthus state. They make their decisions with intuitive confidence, at exactly the right moment. And just as a tightrope walker is always developing his act further, so people in the positive Scleranthus state have the mental capacity for incorporating more and more new potentials into their lives, without losing their balance. Their inner calm, decisiveness and unambiguity has a positive, calming effect on nervous people in their environment.

Scleranthus Key Symptoms
Indecisive; erratic; lacking inner balance. Opinions and moods change from one moment to the next.

Symptoms Due to Energy Block
- Indecisive because of inner restlessness.

- Thoughts constantly vacillating between two possible ways.

- Extreme fluctuation of mood: crying and laughing, in seventh heaven or as miserable as hell.

- A grasshopper mind.

- Seems unreliable because of variable opinions.

- Lack of equilibrium and inner balance, nervous breakdowns.

- Unconcentrated, jumping from topic to topic in conversation.

- Inner lack of decision costs valuable time, with many good opportunities missed both privately and professionally.

- Fails to ask advice of others when in inner conflict, tries to come to decision by oneself.

- Often dithery, jerky gestures.

- Physical symptoms arising from lack of energy balance can be:
  Extreme alternation of activity and apathy, body temperature rising and falling quickly; alternating between hunger and loss of appetite or between constipation and diarrhoea; travel sickness, early morning sickness etc.

Potential Following Transformation
- Power of concentration and determination.

- Maintains inner balance whatever the circumstances.

- Versatile and flexible; able to integrate more and more potentials in one's life.

- Correct decisions are instantaneously made.

- One's presence is soothing to others.

Supportive Measures
- No exaggeration, avoiding extremes; instead of mental zig-zag line, aim for gentle wave motion.

- Breathing exercises to centre oneself and establish a steady pace.

Positive Statements for Practice
'I am finding my own rhythm.'

'The definite decision is to be found within me.'

'I am taking the middle road.'

'I am connected to my Higher Self.'

29. STAR OF BETHLEHEM,
Ornithogalum umbellatum

This plant is related to the onion and to garlic. It grows to a height of 15 or 30cm, its slender leaves showing a white line running down the centre, and may be found in woodlands and meadows. The flowers are striped green on the outside and pure white inside. They will open only when the sun shines, between April and May.

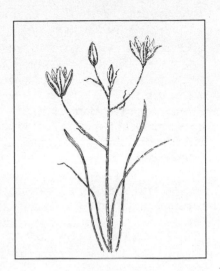

Principle

Star of Bethlehem relates to the soul potentials of awakening and reorientation. A person in the negative Star of Bethlehem state remains in a mental and spiritual half-dream, a kind of inner numbness.

Star of Bethlehem is indicated for all the consequences of physical, mental and spiritual traumatic experiences, irrespective of whether this arose at birth or only yesterday, when one caught a finger in the car door.

Star of Bethlehem is the most important ingredient of Rescue Remedy, synthesizing the actions of the other four Flower Remedies. It will neutralize any form of 'energetic trauma', rapidly restoring the self-healing mechanisms of the body.

Trauma means any direct energy impact that our energetic system is unable to cope with, reacting to it with distortion, irrespective of whether such distortion has been registered by the personality or not. Every 'energetic trauma' will always live on in the energetic system, causing a certain degree of paralysis in the area under its influence.

Practically everybody experiences greater or lesser shocking experience in the course of life that he is unable to cope with. Some shocks will immediately show physical effects. There was the beautician, for instance, who was given notice to vacate her business premises within twenty-four hours. From that moment, she was unable to hear properly, until she was given Star of Bethlehem.

Other traumatic experiences can manifest months or years later as different 'psychosomatic' conditions. Every personality will react individually, in its particular organic weak point.

The negative Star of Bethlehem state does not generally appear as a chronic trait. People in whom this is the case, will often seem slightly drugged and somewhat subdued. They often speak in a low voice that will become even more inaudible towards the end of each sentence. They move slowly and sometimes are subtly inclined towards magic and mysticism. There are many indications that these people carry a karmic burden, with magic, misused ambition and drug abuse playing a role.

As to the source of error in the negative Star of Bethlehem state, this lies in an inner refusal on the part of the personality to take an active part in life.

Rather than play the role on the stage of life that the Higher Self has assigned to the personality it withdraws from everything it does not want to have feelings about, 'battens down the hatches', playing dead, as it were. The result is that a great deal of undigested material collects, clogging the more subtle sensibilities, in fact sometimes more or less poisoning them, so that it gets more and more difficult for information to be conveyed from one energy level to another. The consequence is that even the least energy requirement will be too much for the system, paralysing it; and there will be more and more component areas that can no longer properly come into play.

Bach called Star of Bethlehem 'the comforter and soother of pains and sorrows'.

Star of Bethlehem rouses the personality from its mental half-sleep, taking it back to its Higher Self. It vitalizes energetic links, particularly in the sphere of the nerves. Residues can be dissolved. The personality becomes integrated at all levels; becomes more lively and is able to cope again with normal energy demands. It becomes aware of great vitality, mental clarity and inner strength.

Star of Bethlehem is much used in daily practice, the reason being that no one today escapes traumatic events. This Flower Remedy, and also Holly and Wild Oat, should be considered when there has been no real response to treatment so far. There may be an unconscious shock lodged in the system, blocking everything. Star of Bethlehem acts as a catalyst in this case.

With psychosomatic conditions that prove treatment-resistant, Star of Bethlehem could give quite remarkable results. For example it has often shown to have a relaxing effect when there is tension in the throat or nervous problems with swallowing, i.e. with shocks that have stuck in the throat. Symptoms such as being unable to see, to hear, to walk, to touch, may also be indications for Star of Bethlehem.

People who have taken many narcotics in their life may benefit from Star of Bethlehem combined with Crab Apple.

For the newborn, Star of Bethlehem maybe given to counteract the trauma of birth, together with Walnut for the change to a new form of existence. Some practitioners suggest adding the mixture to the bath water.

Treatments designed to work through psychic traumas, rebirthing for instance, can derive valuable support from Star of Bethlehem.

Star of Bethlehem Key Symptoms
After effects of physical, mental or psychic frightening experiences, irrespective whether of recent to distant origin. 'Comforter and soother of pains and sorrows.'

Symptoms Due to Energy Block
- Unhappy, sad, paralysing sorrow following disappointments, bad news, accidents and other shocking events. The event may be traced back to childhood, and it may also be unconscious. The situation may call for comfort, but one is unable to accept comforting.

- May be inclined towards magic and mysticism.

- Possibly lack of sensation, uncertain gait, tailing off in speech.

- May be taken into consideration as a helper for psychosomatic conditions of all kinds that resist treatment.

- May have history of drug abuse.

Potential Following Transformation
- Inner vitality, clear mind and inner strength.

- Able to adapt nervous system well to energy changes.

- Faculty for quick recovery.

Supportive Measures
Not applicable in the acute stage, but for late sequelae the following may be considered:
- Lymph drainage.

- Therapies designed to work out energetic traumas, e.g. rebirthing.

- Take care of kidneys.

Positive Statements for Practice
'I am letting all energy blocks go.'

'My whole system is breathing.'

'My head is bright and clear.'

'Within me there is total communication.'

30. SWEET CHESTNUT,
Castanea sativa

This tree grows to a height of about 20 metres in open woodlands, in loose soils with a moderate degree of moisture. The catkin-like, sickly scented flowers only appear after the leaves, in June to August, later than on other trees.

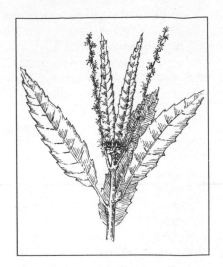

Principle

Sweet Chestnut is connected with the principle of release. A person in the negative Sweet Chestnut state has arrived at a point where he is convinced that there is no more hope nor help for him.

Bach wrote about Sweet Chestnut: 'It is the one (Remedy) for that terrible, that appalling mental despair when it seems the very soul itself is suffering destruction. It is the hopeless despair of those who feel they have reached the limit of their endurance.'

Considering the intensity of suffering, Sweet Chestnut is probably one of the most strongly negative soul states. Yet again it does not always present itself in as dramatic a form as described above, frequently occurring more on inner planes, largely unconscious as far as the person involved is concerned.

The negative Sweet Chestnut state is the moment when the personality is completely on its own, back to the wall, as it were, feeling utterly helpless and unprotected, like a young bird that has fallen from the nest. One hangs suspended in empty space, like a parachutist who has pulled the ripcord a number of times, to no avail. One has fought on uncomplainingly, in courage and hope, but has now come to the end, standing there with empty hands. There is no more yesterday or tomorrow, merely a completely empty, desperate present. One knows that it can only be a matter of hours before the gale-driven flood tide tops the dyke.

The negative Sweet Chestnut state is the moment of truth, the extreme confrontation of the personality with itself and at the same time its last — erroneous — attempt to fight and resist a crucial inner change. It is the night which has to be if day is to rise again.

The intensity of the suffering seems to go beyond what can be borne, the limits of endurance are pushed out farther and farther. This happens so that all the old fixed structures in the personality may be broken up and abandoned, to make room for new dimensions of consciousness.

Sweet Chestnut always initiates new stages of development, e.g. release from a destructive relationship of long standing. The Sweet Chestnut state will often also be the Guardian of the Threshold at the beginning of genuine spiritual development. The human being learns what it really means to be lonely, understanding that only by thus being totally thrown back upon oneself can the way open up to another level of consciousness or to God. One realizes that everything is taken from one because one needs to go forward empty handed if one is to be able to take hold of the new life that is coming towards one; that one has to give oneself up completely to be totally reborn.

Help is nearest when the need is greatest, as the saying goes, and this aptly describes the Sweet Chestnut action. The positive Sweet Chestnut state is one of trust in God, however great the adversity, the moment when cries for help are heard and miracles may happen. Sweet Chestnut helps us to get through difficult periods of transformation, without losing ourselves or getting broken in the process.

People who are in the negative Sweet Chestnut state are always making efforts, similar to Agrimony, to hide their inner despair from others. Even at times of extreme depression they would never think of wanting to put an end to it all, the way Cherry Plum people may do.

As a result, it is not always easy in practice to recognize a negative Sweet Chestnut state. Phrases such as 'I'm at my wit's end', or 'Now I really have no idea how this shall go on' are clear indications.

Differentiating the depressive experience of Gentian, Mustard and Sweet Chestnut:

Gentian	Discouraged through lack of faith; cause is known.
Mustard	Low mood comes and goes like a black cloud, cause not known.
Sweet Chestnut	Deepest mental anguish and despair; acute emergency state for the soul.

Sweet Chestnut Key Symptoms

Feelings of absolute dejection. Thinks one has reached the limits of endurance.

Symptoms Due to Energy Block

- Back to the wall feeling.

- Feeling that utmost limit of endurance has been reached.

- Feels utterly lost inside, helpless in emptiness and total isolation.

- Extreme despair, but no thought of suicide.

- 'Dark night of the soul'.

- No more thought of yesterday or tomorrow; there appears to be nothing but chaos and destruction around one.

- All hope abandoned (more acute than with Gorse), but keeps it to oneself.

- Afraid one may break down under the stress against one's will.

Potential Following Transformation

- Experience of nothingness on the threshold to new horizons.

- Was lost and has found oneself again.

- Phoenix rising from the ashes.

- Has recognized that a crucial change is possible, the inner journey has started.

- Able to believe again, personal experiences of God.

Supportive Measures

- Consider the idea of having to learn through pain on this planet, and the concept of salvation.

- Recreation in the light and in unspoiled nature.

Positive Statements for Practice
'Night has to come before it can be day again.'

'Through darkness to light.'

'When the need is greatest, God's help is nearest.'

'My inner self is inviolable.'

31. VERVAIN,
Verbena officinalis

A robust upright perennial,
vervain may be found by the
roadside, on dry, waste
ground and in sunny
pastures. The small lilac or
mauve coloured flowers
open between July and
September.

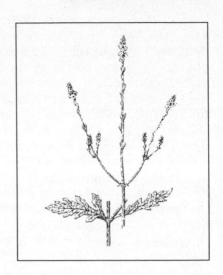

Principle

Vervain relates to the soul potentials of self-discipline and restraint. In the negative Vervain state the will is directed too much to the outside, and energies are not used economically and therefore squandered.

On a school trip, young Peter has been asked by his teacher to keep reminding him of the time, so that the programme may run smoothly. Bursting with pride at having been given the responsibility he sets about the task with great eagerness. He gets up thinking of the time, he goes to sleep thinking of it, and if he wakes in the night his first thought is what time it may be. He wants to do the job not a hundred but a hundred and fifty per cent, almost outdoing himself. His teacher only has to look at him and he'll be bursting to say what time it is. If the other boys and girls are dawdling he will run after them, almost begging them to hurry up, surely they must know how important it is to be punctual. Young Peter finds no relaxation on this class trip. He is on the job all the time and his classmates end up by calling him 'the clock'; an early example of a Vervain type.

An inner flame is aglow in Vervain people, usually a positive idea that fills them utterly, and they are quite unable to rest until everybody else around them has also become convinced of the idea. Chairmen and chairwomen of welfare organizations, sacrificing their free time and many night time hours to the 'good cause', never fearing to say what has to be said, are Vervain types. They are always on call, feeling dedicated to their role, like actors. With missionary zeal they will try to win over everybody they meet for the cause, sometimes successfully, sometimes not. The reason is that in their eagerness they overdo things, always the passionate protagonist, bombarding the other person with their arguments, and not so much the skilled diplomat who will let the other have his say as well.

With such an excessive use of will-power they tend to overdraw on their energy account. They are tense and nervous inside and out, and react angrily when things are not progressing as well as they expected. As a result they get even more involved, trying to take even more out of themselves. They'll never allow themselves a free minute throughout the day, and only have a few hours sleep at night. They overestimate their vital energy and carry on regardless of their health. Suddenly they'll 'catch the 'flu', their immune system having been weakened.

Some people are so keyed up when in the negative Vervain state that, even if they wanted to, they would find it difficult to relax physically. Their muscle tension is colossal, as may be noted from their expressive demeanour and the way physical activities, too, are carried out with an excess of energy. They will grip a pencil so hard, for instance, that it almost breaks, and when they come up the stairs it sounds as though they were wearing army boots.

Vervain types radiate their energy and unlike Rock Water types sometimes want to convince others in a missionary way. They are revolutionaries at heart, 'going to the barricades in their just anger', sometimes not even noticing that they are triggering off a whole avalanche of complications. They are 'itinerant preachers' at heart, people conscious of their mission, people who 'can never keep their mouth shut' and are prepared to go to prison for their convictions. In the extreme case it may also be the student who pours petrol over himself and sets fire to himself in public. Unfortunately these people are often doing more harm than good for their cause, for they are quickly written off as fanatics. This is the tragedy and the error in the negative Vervain state.

A person in the negative vervain state has heard the call

from his soul and wants to follow it. He will therefore be flooded with a great deal of positive energy at times, with the personality and the body as yet unable to cope. The personality will make efforts to utilize this energy, but still lacks knowledge of certain laws and experience in dealing with large volumes of positive energy. The personality takes hold of this energy and tries to 'make' something of it on the basis of its own limited concepts, rather than simply letting it act on its own. It is attempting, as it were, to force a strong jet of water through a hose that is too narrow.

The personality has to learn that it has not been given this energy to squander indiscriminately, as it sees fit, but has to 'turn its money to account'. This also means looking after the body which is the vessel for those energies, and not play fast and loose with it. Another thing it has to realize is that pressure will always produce counterpressure, and that there is no need for a 'hard sell' with a good idea, for it is much more convincing if one embodies the idea, if one 'is' the idea.

A person in the positive Vervain state has practised and learned to master his divine unrest and use his energies with love, but effectively. He will be wholly involved in his task, but also be prepared at all times to hear the opinions of others and review his own position if necessary. He will think in a wider context. With his exuberant character he is able to inspire others and carry them along easily.

The key difference between Vine and Vervain:

Vervain Wants to enthuse others with his ideas, and in his excessive eagerness uses too much pressure.

Vine Deliberately uses a lot of pressure to achieve his own egotistical ends.

Vervain Key Symptoms
Over enthusiastic in supporting a good cause. Strains his energies; highly-strung and even fanatical.

Symptoms Due to Energy Block
- Enthusiastic about an idea, wants to carry others along.

- Has firm principles, rarely deviating from them, and always wanting to convince others as to their rightness.

- Very intense, focusing too strongly, wants to achieve one hundred and fifty per cent.

- Impulsive, idealistic, even fancifully so.

- Great consciousness of mission, always on the job.

- Tells others how to do things in one's overeagerness, acting for them, trying to force them into what is good for them.

- Wants to convert others, absolutely drowning them in one's energy, tiring them out.

- Overdoes things, gets ahead of oneself; wants to 'sell' an idea to others, and does not serve the cause with this.

- Does a subject to death; fanatic.

- Incensed by injustices.

- Courageous, accepting risks, prepared to make sacrifices to achieve one's goals.

- Uses enormous energies to keep going, even when physical strength is exhausted.

- Irritable and nervous, 'nerves raw', when things do not progress as well as expected.

- Tends to be wiry type, speaks and moves swiftly.

- Living on one's nerves, liable to states of exhaustion and nervous breakdowns.

- Totally keyed up, quite unable to relax; often suffers from muscle tension, pain in eyes, headaches, etc.

- Hyperactive children who can't be got to bed at night.

Potential Following Transformation
- Stands up for one's ideas, but also gives others the right to have their own opinions.

- May allow oneself to be converted to another view by good arguments in a discussion.

- Sees things in a wider context.

- Able to use one's great energies effectively and with love for a worthwhile end.

- The 'torch bearer', effortlessly able to enthuse and inspire others, and to carry them along.

Supportive Measures

- Understand that any system will break down some time or other if constant tension is applied, and that this will serve no one.

- Accept that it is not always the intensity of the effort put in, but adaptable psychological tactics that will lead to success.

- Do not 'over-ride' the other person but 'ride with him'.

- Make room for specific breaks for relaxation in the day's programme: sit down, do breathing exercises, etc.

- Tai Chi and other forms of meditation involving slow, harmonious movement.

- Competitive sport or dance lessons, to channel the energies and powers of concentration in a positive way.

Positive Statements for Practice

'I am holding back, letting the others come on.'

'I am harmonizing my energies, to use them with more care and to better effect.'

'I am becoming a vessel for higher powers, and wholly give myself up to inner guidance.'

32. VINE,
Vitis vinifera

A climbing plant, growing to
a length of 15 metres or
more, the vine grows in
countries with warmer
climates. The small, fragrant
green flowers grow in dense
clusters. The flowering time
varies with the climate.

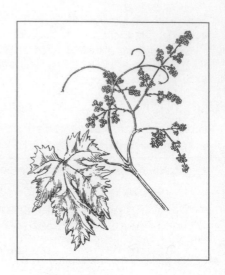

Principle
Vine relates to the soul potential of authority and ability to
carry conviction. A person in the extreme negative Vine state
is hard, greedy for power, with no respect for the
individuality of others.

Vine is a very powerful form of energy, giving a person
above-average leadership qualities whilst at the same time
also making extreme demands on his personality. There is a
tremendous temptation to let oneself be hypnotized by this
volcanic force, using it only to satisfy limited, egotistical
ends.

Vine types are very capable, ambitious and unsurpassed
when it comes to will-power and presence of mind. They will
find a way out of every crisis situation, and always hold the
reins; in the struggle for survival they will always be
victorious, familiar with success. Sooner or later this will lead
to a conviction of being infallible, and they will think that
they are in fact doing others a favour in telling them how to
do things, insisting that it is done their way.

'I can't see what they are on about. It's in their own interest
...', the authoritarian head of the department says to a
colleague who is trying to suggest that his leadership style is
somewhat too militaristic. 'They haven't got a clue anyway',
he will say and shaking his head get on with the day's work.
The next time sales figures are assessed his department again
comes out best, and he wonders if he should not use the

opportunity to take over his colleague's department as well. Human regard — fairness? — ridiculous! 'Business is business, and you have to be ruthless if necessary.'

Many evildoers, villains and tyrants in history were negative Vine types. Open any newspaper today and the reports on dictatorships, cruelty and torture make it quite clear that negative Vine energy is still wreaking the same havoc on our planet to this very day.

A person in the negative Vine state loses all feeling for other people, falling victim to his own powerful ideas: 'The boy needs to be handled roughly', a father will say, accepting the fact that his son will lose all affection for him and only fear him. 'You are not supposed to think, just do exactly what I say ...' the strict old ballet teacher is saying, swinging the baton in her fingers. People in need of Vine include a surprisingly high proportion of artists who are highly sensitive and extremely ambitious, forcing themselves to train every day, with iron discipline, always worried at the back of their minds about their condition, the first-night date and anxiety as to their careers. This anxiety, coupled with ambition, an iron will and a compulsion to be successful, forms the conflict that lies behind practically every negative Vine state.

It reveals the error of the personality, which lies in using the tremendous forces flowing towards it — forces it certainly is not always able entirely to cope with — only for its own benefit, to satisfy its own vanity, rather than place them in the service of a higher plan. 'What benefit is it to you to be a demigod, unless you are a divine being?' An American spiritualist asked this question, and it applies particularly to people with strong Vine traits.

When we take Vine, opening up to our Higher Self and to the higher goals of the soul, we will realize that we are supported by the very power that we were trying to use to gain control over everything before. We will feel how will-power unites with love, and strength with wisdom. When our actions are no longer entirely egotistical, but done in relation to the greater whole, new strength will come as though of its own accord.

We become the instrument of a higher plane, and our actions will then also automatically serve the positive interests of our fellow men. Their conscious or unconscious recognition will give new energies to positive Vine types, lending them a natural authority, without need for an imperious air.

A person in the positive Vine state will realize that 'strong leadership qualities' are in fact only needed in temporary crisis situations, and that most of the time one is merely 'the first servant of the country', as the German king Frederic the Great put it so aptly. He will feel his function to be to help others find their own way.

In practice, the Vine state very often appears together with other, weaker soul states: Mimulus for example, Pine, Larch or Centaury. The conflict in the personality may, for instance, lie in a very impressionable nature (Centaury) needing to be compensated for by will-power and hardness (Vine).

The negative Vine state may be found with all physical conditions giving expression to powerful inner tensions. Women in the Vine state are role-conscious, which is mostly hidden. The iron will and demanding nature is seldom expressed verbally, but rather through gestures, glances and actions.

Vine Key Symptoms
Dominating, inflexible, striving for power.

Symptoms Due to Energy Block
- Very capable, extremely sure of oneself, extreme will-power.

- Ambitious and presumptuous.

- Thinks one knows exactly what is right for others; everybody has to dance to one's tune.

- The man or woman who with presence of mind and firm decision saves the situation; good leaders.

- Runs the risk of misusing one's great gifts for personal ambitions of power.

- Disregards the opinions of others, demanding absolute obedience.

- Greedy for power, wants authority, aggressive, no scruples in choosing one's methods.

- Never doubts one's superiority for a second, and

therefore imposes one's will on others.

- The domestic tyrant, the stern father, the dictator.
- Disposition hard, ruthless, even cruel, with no pangs of conscience.
- Governs by consciously putting fear into others.
- Even on one's sickbed will tell the physician what he ought to do, keeping the nursing staff on the run.
- Refuses to discuss things, because one is right anyway.
- People refusing to join in the power game are ignored.
- May toady to superiors and bully subordinates.
- Unyielding inside, resulting in extreme inner tension and possible painful physical conditions.
- Children who bully their playmates.

Potential Following Transformation
- Wise, understanding leader; beloved teacher who has natural authority; 'good shepherd'.
- Able to delegate and place one's leadership qualities in the service of a greater task.
- Helps others to help themselves and find their own way.

Supportive Measures
- Teamwork — practise being one among many.
- In conversation, seek communion with the Higher Self of the other person.
- Yoga exercises to harmonize the energy field.
- Tai Chi, to experience the flow of energy.

Postitive Statements for Practice
'To rule is to serve.'

'I recognize and respect the unique nature of every individual.'

'I give help towards self-help.'

'Your will be done.'

33. WALNUT,
Juglans regia

This tree grows to a height
of up to 30 metres and does
well in protected areas, by
hedges and in orchards.
Male and female flowers
grow on the same tree, the
male ones in much greater
number than the greeny
females. The tree blooms in
April or May, before or just
as the leaf-buds burst.

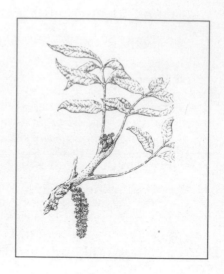

Principle
Walnut relates to the soul qualities of a new beginning and of
unaffectedness. A person in the Walnut state finds it hard to
take that final step, some negative aspects of his personality
still being caught up, consciously or unconsciously, in old
decisions or the bonds of the past.

Just as our forefathers venerated the walnut as a regal tree,
the Walnut Flower Remedy also holds a special position
among the 38 Bach Flowers. It is needed mostly in special life
situations where major changes are about to take place. Such
situations may be conversion to a new faith, entering a
convent, changing to a completely different occupation,
emigrating to another country.

Walnut thus helps with new beginnings in the mental and
spiritual sphere, but it also proves useful in major stages of
biological change. These, too, mean vital inner changes and
liberate completely new energy potentials — in teething for
instance, puberty, pregnancy, the menopause, or in the
terminal stages of physical life.

All situations involving major change are phases of
increased stress, and therefore of increased inner instability.
In periods of this kind, even stable characters who normally
know very well what they want are inclined to vacillate. They
are apt to listen to the suggestive warnings and scepticism of
others, fall back into old habits, get caught up in sentimental

musings, conventional ideas or old family traditions, running the risk of abandoning their inner decision.

A person in the negative Walnut state is mentally sitting in a boat that is to take him across the river. He can clearly see the opposite bank, but the boat is still partly tied up. The last of the ropes are still keeping him unconsciously tied to the past, perhaps an unexpected unpleasant experience, a relationship to a partner that has not been digested, perhaps even a decision one is not even aware of. All that is needed is that final, decisive push, the captain giving the command to cast off.

Bach wrote that Walnut is 'the Remedy for those who have decided to take a great step forward in life, to break old conventions, to leave old limits and restrictions and start on a new way.' Such a farewell to old relationships, thoughts and feelings is always painful and may frequently also express itself physically.

The Walnut state is normally only temporary, and genuine Walnut types are not too common nowadays. When we do meet one, he'll be something of a pioneer, often ahead of others in fighting for certain ideals and ideas. These are the people who are innovators in the sphere of ideas. They have firmly defined life goals, sometimes tending to be rather unconventional in bringing them to realization. Yet being open at heart, they may face a temporary risk of losing their original direction though pressure from others.

They are, however, only able to fulfil their mission if left quite unhampered in soul and spirit, and therefore have to shake off anything that might tie them down. Walnut* will provide the support and firmness they need for this.

If we may speak of an error of the personality in the negative Walnut state, this lies in temporarily losing unaffectedness, and in a delayed reaction to the impulses of the Higher Self. Whilst open to inner guidance, a person in this state still allows himself to be distracted too easily, rather than submitting fully to the guidance of his Higher Self. The personality will still take its lead from other people and ideas

---

*It is interesting that a walnut kernel and the cerebrum show very similar convolutions. The present view is that decisions are made in the cerebral cortex.

at times, when they should be concentrating on the task set by their own soul.

The reasons for this often lie far back, in other forms of existence. They may be karmic bonds that have not yet been recognized, wrong decisions made long ago that are having an autosuggestive effect at the unconscious level. Bach therefore also called Walnut the 'breaker of spells'. Walnut energy forms a bridge between different planes, creating an inner link between destiny unfolding in front of the curtain and behind it. It helps to achieve final release from the shadows and fetters of the past.

A person in the positive Walnut state is completely free in spirit, able to set sail for new horizons. He makes progress in fulfilling his life mission, unaffected by outer circumstances and the opinions of others. Edward Bach himself was an example of the positive Walnut type. In the last years of his life, he let go of everything — social approval, financial security, the traditions of orthodox medicine, his whole past professional life. Despite wry looks from his former colleagues, he followed the call he had received, in the most modest financial circumstances.

Some examples of stages of progressive change where Walnut has been found helpful in practice, usually in combination with other character-specific Flower Remedies are as follows:

On starting retirement; on voluntarily moving to an old people's home; following a stroke or other illness that means a major change in life style; on starting work, entering into a world that is very different from one's home background; after psychotherapy, when completely new elements of the personality have become accessible, leading to new inner decisions; during divorce proceedings, when physical separation has already taken place, but something still ties one to the former partner and his or her negative thoughts are still liable to make their mark.

Some practitioners use Walnut to screen themselves from their patients' energy radiations. It has also been used to fix the energies of high potency homoeopathic treatment and in the treatment of addiction, particularly nicotine addiction. The Remedy has also been found to have a stabilizing effect with chiropractic manipulation of the spine and with dental problems.

Differentiating between different Bach Flower Remedies as regards openness to influence and indecision:

Centaury	Easily influenced because own will is weak.
Cerato	Easily influenced because one does not trust one's own judgement.
Scleranthus	Easily influenced because of total lack of mental focus; is all the time torn to and fro at energy level.
Wild Oat	Easily influenced because ambitions not definite.
Honeysuckle	Easily influenced because mind largely dwelling on the past.
Clematis	Easily influenced because mind tends to dwell in fantasy world.
Walnut	Easily influenced because of increased sensitivity and instability during important phases of new beginnings in life.

Walnut Key Symptoms
Difficulties of adjusting in transition periods of life. Wants to resist powerful influences and follow one's own true ambitions.

Symptoms Due to Energy Block
- Normally knows exactly what one wants, but now tends to vacillate in a specific new situation.

- Has made a major decision affecting one's life, only the last step remains to be taken.

- Finally wants to leave behind all restrictions and influences, but does not quite succeed.

- Finds it hard to escape the influence of a dominant personality when making decisions relating to one's own life — parents, partners, teachers, etc.

- An unexpected outside event forces one to rethink one's whole approach to life.

- Crucial changes occur in life: change of occupation, divorce, retirement, move to another town, move to an old people's home, etc.

- Major biological changes are about to occur: menopause,

pregnancy, puberty, teething, terminal stages of illness.

- Finally wants to be really clear in one's mind concerning a change.

- Has given up a relationship, but despite physical separation still feels under the old partner's spell.

Potential Following Transformation
- The pioneer who remains true to himself.

- Follows one's life goal undeviatingly, despite adverse circumstances, and not influenced by others.

- Open and unprejudiced towards anything new.

- Recognizes the laws behind the changes which occur.

- Is immune to outside influence and open to inner inspiration.

- Able at last to free oneself from the shadows of the past.

Supportive Measures
- During periods of change: get enough sleep, eat sensibly. Avoid any additional factors that might cause further uncertainty and instability for the personality.

- Meditate on the Crown chakra.

- Contemplate the principles and mode of action of great masters.

Positive Statements for Practice
'I am only following my own inner guidance.'

'I dismiss all limiting factors that stop me from reaching my life's goal.'

'I am holding out.'

'Destructive influences pass me by.'

34. WATER VIOLET,
Hottonia palustris

This is a member of the primrose family, flowering in May and June in slow moving or stagnant water, pools and ditches. The pale lilac flowers with their yellow centres grow in whorls around the leafless stalk. The finely divided leaves remain below the surface of the water.

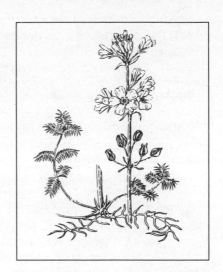

Principle

Water Violet relates to the soul qualities of humility and wisdom. A person in the negative Water Violet state is not behaving as wisely as he might, withdrawing in proud reserve.

Water Violet energy often represents itself in a largely transformed quality so that the negative Water Violet traits show themselves in conjunction with the positive Water Violet potential, being temporary deviations as it were.

The appearance of the plant provides a good illustration of its essential energy: delicate but upright. The part giving stability to the plant, the leaves, stay below the surface of the water.

People with strong Water Violet traits are usually well in control of their highly developed personality. They present an image of unobtrusive superiority and calm sovereignty. In the eyes of others, they may therefore appear unapproachable and unassailable. Water Violet types are different from others. Like a well bred Siamese cat, they move silently in space, with dignified delicacy, choosing their own way, not influenced by others. Seeing such a creature, many of us must have thought: 'that's how I should like to be!' Yet despite their above-average abilities and high degree of individuality, Water Violet characters also have their own very special problems.

Take the much admired yoga teacher. In spite of her sovereign manner and superior qualities, she sometimes feels isolated from her fellows. She does not find it easy, on those days, to step down from the pedestal on which her students have placed her, and approach them with ease. Gushing, rather emotive camaraderie is not her style, her affection has more spiritual roots, and she sometimes does not know how far she should go in her heart, and in case of doubt tends to show reserve. Others find it difficult to break through her highly personal sound barrier, yet Water Violet types are always asked for advice, and often made into a kind of emotional dustbin.

When the drain on the energy due to the demands of others gets too great, it may happen quite suddenly that Water Violet types, inwardly shaking their heads, will come to the conclusion that they really seem to be something special, and lapse into their inherited fault of pride and superciliousness, withdrawing into their tortoise shell. There they are not to be disturbed. Just as on principle they do not interfere in their affairs of others, so they reject third-party interference in their affairs, even when ill. They prefer to deal with their own problems. They like to keep a stiff upper lip even when on their own, and this blocks much of their energy, in the long run maybe leading to tension and stiffness in the whole body.

People with marked Water Violet traits are much appreciated as superiors, not only because they are conscientious in their work, but particularly because they have the ability to be something of a calm, objective rock in the roaring surf of departmental emotions. They are almost always on top of things, but prefer to use tact in their work and actions, calmly, from the background. The only thing they find difficult is to make harsh decisions, for they are always aware of the situation of everybody involved. Unlike Vine, a Water Violet boss will never force an employee to do something. But if his wishes do not penetrate for a long time, he will inwardly withdraw from that person.

A person in the negative Water Violet state who remains too long within his tortoise shell is not doing himself a favour, for he is isolating himself from the living exchange of energies without which even the most sovereign amongst us are unable to exist. The personality gets more and more frozen in relation to its environment and also to itself. It has turned away from its Higher Self at this moment, wrongly so, and refuses to acknowledge that its superiority and special qualities are also an obligation.

Rather than shutting himself off from others in his separateness, the Water Violet personality should pass on his values in conscious or unconscious energy exchanges with others, and in his superiority be an inspiring example.

This exemplary element is an outstanding trait of people in the positive Water Violet state. They are an island of peace, calm and confidence for those around them. They progress through life with kind grace and inner dignity.

Teachers and people working in the healing professions are often Water Violet types. When one gets the temporary feeling, as a therapist, of being unable to make contact with one's patients, or suddenly feels the need to withdraw completely from the world, Water Violet is indicated.

In some very interesting cases, a symbolic eczema developed on the right hand of these therapists. That is the hand with which we reach out into the world.

Water Violet Key Symptoms
Inner reserve, proud withdrawal, feeling of superiority in isolation, little emotional involvement.

Symptoms Due to Energy Block
- Sometimes feels isolated because of one's superiority.

- Being out of the ordinary, sometimes appears reserved, and will then be considered conceited or supercilious.

- Will not permit others to interfere in one's life.

- Sorts things out for oneself, won't burden others with one's problems.

- Wants to be left alone when unwell.

- Sometimes finds it difficult to approach others with ease.

- At times wants to withdraw completely, 'my home is my castle'.

- Others find it difficult to break through the 'sound barrier' and make genuine personal contact.

- Avoids disputes with emotional overtones, as one finds them exhausting.

- Dislikes having to make harsh decisions, always being able to see the situation of everybody involved.

- Is much sought after for advice.

- Rarely cries, endeavours to keep stiff upper lip.

Potential Following Transformation
- Charming, gentle, showing tactful reserve.

- Independent attitude, equable, on the calm side.

- Capable, competent, often superior to others.

- Self-confidence, knows who one is.

- Comfortable with oneself, likes to be on one's own.

- Generally has life well in hand.

- Moves quietly, beautifully and unobtrusively.

- Often speaks in a low, polite and insistent voice.

- Tolerant attitude — live and let live.

- Would never interfere, even if one sees things quite differently.

- Usually on top of things, 'rock in the foaming waves'.

- Works in sovereign fashion, conscientiously, prefers to stay in the background.

- For others the image of a well-balanced, independent-minded person.

- Acts in humility, love and wisdom.

- Able to create an atmosphere of calm, confidence and tranquillity.

- Goes through life with elegance and inner dignity.

Supportive Measures
- Train oneself to attune consciously to the Higher Selves of all who one is dealing with.

- Take up 'earth-bound' creative hobbies.

Positive Statements for Practice
'I am part, I take part.'

'I need the world and the world needs me.'

'I am sharing love, humility and wisdom.'

35. WHITE CHESTNUT,
Aesculus hippocastanum

This is the horse chestnut, flowering at the end of May or in early June. The male flowers tend to be at the top of the 'candelabra', the female lower down. The colour of the flowers is creamy white splashed and dotted with crimson and yellow.

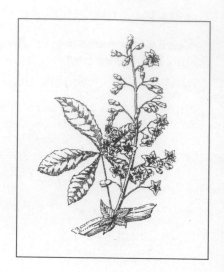

Principle

White Chestnut relates to the soul qualities of tranquillity and discernment. A person in the negative White Chestnut state is the victim of misunderstood, unsuitable mental concepts.

We all know the state when there has been trouble at work. After two hours of hot debate everything seems to be settled to satisfaction.

At night, you are sitting in the bathtub, hoping to relax, but the dispute you had at work still goes on. You are now thinking of everything else you should have said. Over and over again you are defending yourself to an imaginary works committee. Again and again you hear the derogatory remark made by a business partner, and yet you had such a high opinion of him. Surely it cannot be that he is proving such a disappointment to you? Should you sever the connection? But what of the big new order that has just come in? Forget about it, tomorrow morning you can consider it all dispassionately, now its time for bed and a good sleep. But sleep is out of the question. The roundabout of your thoughts continues to go through its gyrations as you lie in bed, with the same arguments and counter arguments. Oh, if only one could turn off those tiresome thoughts, simply stop them.

People showing strong White Chestnut traits do not go through this just once, but frequently. Many have got so used to those dialogues in their mind that they take them more or less for normal.

In the negative White Chestnut state we are victims to an overweaning mental process that has gained the upper hand over all other personality levels. Some people in need of White Chestnut experienced their head as a completely separate energy unit during meditation.

'In my thoughts I am like a hamster in his wheel, not getting a single step further', said a grammar school boy in the White Chestnut state. 'My thoughts are mental earwigs. They simply won't disappear from my head and they have the upper hand completely.' 'The other day I was so busy with my mental arguments I almost drove through a red traffic light.' 'My head is so full of mental chatter that I can't formulate a single clear thought when in the office.' Those, too, are typical statements made by people in the negative White Chestnut state.

Quite a few of them suffer from a chronic frontal headache,* particularly above the eyes. Many have problems in going to sleep, or their thoughts will wake them from their sleep at four in the morning, refusing to go like tiresome door salesmen.

The face will also often betray great mental tension. People in the White Chestnut state tend to unconsciously grind their lower jaws.

In his *Handbook of the Bach Flower Remedies*, Dr Philip Chancellor writes that 'unlike Clematis who uses his thoughts to escape from the world, the White Chestnut type would give anything to escape from his thoughts into the world', to get his brain cool and clear.

There are many different hypotheses as to the origin of the White Chestnut state. Bach himself said that it occurred when the mind wandered from matters in hand, losing concentration and allowing other unresolved and perhaps more important thoughts to come to the surface.

In every case it appears that a process of selection at the level of soul and spirit is not functioning as well as it should. The mind has not developed an ability to discriminate between thoughts and ideas that should be accepted by the system and those that should be rejected. It greedily takes in

---

*Nineteenth century popular medicine advised three raw chestnuts to be carried on one's person for three days to treat a headache due to nervous causes rather than an excess of blood to the head. A successful prescription.

everything that comes, and then finds itself unable to integrate anything.

The ideas flutter about like disarrayed papers on a small writing desk, the unimportant pieces concealing the important documents and generally causing consternation. The only solution is to tidy the writing desk, sorting the important from the unimportant.

In the negative White Chestnut state the personality has turned its back on guidance from its Higher Self, and this shows itself in the consequences of its egotistical, mental greed. In the absence of guidance and orientation on setting a higher goal for life, the personality is playing around with too much thought energy, often misunderstanding, losing the way and falling victim to foreign impulses that have no place in its soul programme. As soon as it once again accepts the guidance of its Higher Self and its soul, all mental impulses are automatically selected to serve its best interests. It can let go of all interfering foreign thought elements that block the view of its own soul programme.

In the positive White Chestnut state, the personality is able to let any foreign thought impulse rush past it like a fast non-stop train, never feeling tempted to get on it. Calm and peace are the keynotes of its mental state. From the clear lake of its consciousness the answers that are wanted and solutions to problems emerge of their own accord. People who are in the positive White Chestnut state are able to make constructive use of their powerful mental plane.

Distinction between Hornbeam, Scleranthus and White Chestnut as regards the feeling of thoughts weighing one down:

Hornbeam	Head heavy, feels mentally overburdened; tiredness predominates.
Scleranthus	Mentally vacillating between two choices, like a grasshopper; less head-orientated than White Chestnut.
White Chestnut	Very much head-orientated; thoughts constantly going round in one's head; prisoner of one's thoughts.

White Chestnut Key Symptoms
Unwanted thoughts keep going round and round in one's head, cannot get rid of them, mental arguments and dialogues.

Symptoms Due to Energy Block
- Unwanted thoughts constantly come to mind, cannot be turned off.

- A worry or event won't let go of one, gnawing on one's mind.

- Again and again thinks of 'what one might have said' or 'should have said'.

- The feeling that a gramophone record keeps jumping its groove.

- Uselessly treading water mentally, feeling like a hamster in his wheel.

- Constant mental chatter, head a hall of echoes.

- Keep going over the same problems time and time again in one's mind.

- Mental hyperactivity, therefore lacks concentration in everyday life (e.g. does not hear when one is being addressed).

- Cannot sleep because of the thoughts going round in one's head, particularly in the early hours of the morning.

- Tired and depressed during the day, head feels full.

- May have frontal headache, eyes hurt.

Potential Following Transformation
- Balanced state of mind.

- Head clear and calm.

- Solution for every problem comes up of its own accord from a calm mind.

- Able to use one's powers of thought constructively.

Supportive Measures
- Reflect on the subject of 'thought power'.

- Resolve unwanted trains of thought by visualization, e.g. dissolve them in water, burn them in the fire, cover them with snow, put them on a railway train etc.

- Breathing exercises, yoga exercises to harmonize the energetic system.

Positive Statements for Practice
'Calm flows right through me.'

'Everything is taking its proper course.'

'The solution I need will be coming to mind of its own accord.'

'I dismiss all strange and outdated thought concepts.'

36. WILD OAT,
Bromus ramosus

A grass commonly found in damp woods, thickets and by roadsides. The hermaphrodite flowers are enclosed by scales in their spikelets.

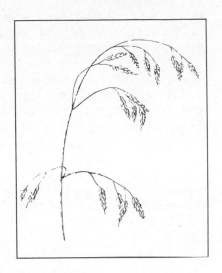

Principle

Wild Oat relates to the soul qualities of vocation and purposefulness. A person in the negative Wild Oat state does not know his true vocation, and therefore feels unfulfilled and dissatisfied in his heart of hearts.

Typical Wild Oat people will often show this trait even in their young days. They are usually richly gifted and need make no special effort to achieve anything. Many things just fall into their lap. Despite this they are ambitious and want to achieve something special. On the other hand they only have a vague notion as to what this may be. At the same time Wild Oat types also want to enjoy life, generally in rather unconventional ways. They don't want to go with the current but steer their own craft. Unfortunately they do not know the name of the port. Wild Oat types therefore also find it difficult to fit into society. They do not like to commit themselves, and it can happen that lack of definition causes them to end up in groups that are not at the same level intellectually or spiritually, resulting in further frustration.

Life is for ever offering new opportunities to Wild Oat types. They will start many things, often have a number of professions and be quite successful at them, but will always lack that real inner certainty that will permit a final, definite decision. After some time, the work that until now has been so enjoyable begins to pall, and in one's heart the colleagues among whom one has felt so much at home are now critically judged rather boring. The Wild Oat type himself tears down what he has built up, to move on to the next opportunity, in the hope that this will prove really satisfactory.

Someone who has had no experience of such things might well imagine that such a state of creative unrest can be most stimulating, but in the long run the opposite is the case. People in the negative Wild Oat state feel life passing them by, in spite of all their talents and activities. They feel regret at never being able to be wholly affirmative, never being able to really enjoy the fruits of their labours.

Wild Oat types are eternal bachelors at heart, always on the look-out and never reaching the goal. Their condition may indeed also be described as delayed mental puberty. The head is full of odd ideas, notions as to all the things one would like to and ought to do. One is still at the stage of sowing one's wild oats, squandering one's energies in all directions, rather than finally accepting the guidance of the Higher Self and going for a single goal.

The error in the negative Wild Oat state is one of excessive selfwilledness and self-centredness of the personality, in blind eagerness in looking for goals and decisions in the outside world, instead of realizing that it merely needs to follow the inner guidance of its Higher Self to discover that the decision, long since made, lies within itself.

People who are in the Wild Oat state need to learn to go for depth rather than breadth. They will find that life does not get more boring, as they thought it might, but on the contrary, offers undreamt of new experiences. With every decision they make they should ask for the real inner reason. For they have to realize that it is not a question of doing something 'special', but to do the right thing in a given situation and to do it as thoroughly and well as possible, since everything we do is an essential part of a greater, meaningful progress. They need to know that their rich talents are needed within the context of the greater whole, and ask for inner guidance.

A person taking Wild Oat will feel himself gradually growing calmer, clearer and more certain in heart and mind. Little by little he will have a clearer picture of what it is he really wants, and will come to act intuitively rather than impulsively. It is possible to firmly align his many different gifts, make them serve a higher goal, and even the most enticing new opportunities that may beckon will not make him let go of the thread he has found. Life continues to offer plenty of variety, but it will now be more fulfilling and happy.

Like Holly, Wild Oat is considered a good opener in a course of treatment, when the combination of Flower Remedies used has not brought a response, or when it seems that too many Flowers are indicated at once.

Wild Oat does, however, also often present as a long-term condition that can be traced right back to childhood. Typical Wild Oat children are rarely members of a gang or similar peer group. They never really take part and are everywhere and nowhere. Sometimes an adulthood Wild Oat state traces back to very domineering parents who never allowed the child to decide for himself, weakening the development of his personality. Wild Oat is always indicated where vocational decisions have to be made and often in male 'midlife crisis'. In the experience of some practitioners, Wild Oat types sometimes have sexual problems. Many are also inclined to eat too much.

The difference between Scleranthus and Wild Oat as regards indecision:

Scleranthus   Vacillates between two polar opposites.
Wild Oat   Has so many opportunities that he often does not even come to the point of choosing between two alternatives.

Wild Oat Key Symptoms
Indefinite as to ambitions, dissatisfaction because one's mission in life is not found.

Symptoms Due to Energy Block
- Has vague notions as to aims, cannot find direction in life. This leads to dissatisfaction, frustration and boredom.

- Is ambitious, wants to do something special, but does not know exactly what.

- Though ambitious, does not feel inclined towards any particular profession and such 'hanging in the air' leads to despondency.

- Is depressed because things are not as clear-cut for one as for others.

- Has many gifts, tries out all kinds of things, but finds no real satisfaction.

- Unchannelled talents and abilities.

- Does not want to commit oneself, and because of this unconsciously tends to end up in the same unsatisfactory situations again and again.

- Easily dissipates one's gifts and energies.

- Does not know where one fits in.

- Professional or private life is not of the right kind.

Potential Following Transformation
- Ability to recognize one's potential and develop it to the full.

- Wide range of talents; one is able to follow a higher guideline and always bring things to completion.

- Has clear ideas and ambitions and will not allow oneself to be deflected.

- Able to do many things well, even successfully do several jobs simultaneously.

Supportive Measures
- Begin to make life subject to higher, spiritual goals.

- Ask for spiritual guidance.

- Establish a scale of values for different interests, pursuing some as hobbies and using others professionally.

- Begin to plan only in the mid-term, but bring everything to full completion.

Positive Statements for Practice
'I am following the predestined course in my life.'

'I am accepting inner guidance.'

'I am putting my talents to the service of the greater whole.'

37. WILD ROSE,
Rosa canina

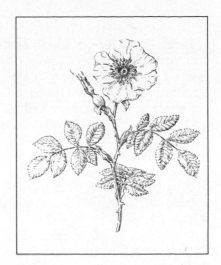

The ancestor of many cultivated roses, the wild rose likes to grow in the sun, on the fringes of woods, in hedgerows and on stony slopes. The flowers are white, pale pink or deep pink, with five large heart-shaped petals. They open singly or in groups of three between June and August.

Principle

Wild Rose relates to the soul potentials of devotion and inner motivation. A person in the negative Wild Rose state misunderstands the principle of devotion and takes it negatively.

In the Wild Rose state, one is not happily going along with life, devoted to one's task within the greater whole, but instead lives in extremely fixed, personality-linked negative expectations. The misunderstanding often arises during the first days of life, or it may possibly derive from earlier forms of existence. As a result, personal initiative is completely abandoned, and there is apathetic resignation with regard to inner and outer life.

A baby that has been crying for its mother for hours will at some point give up hope of its mother ever coming to relieve its hunger. Feeling utterly deserted and in complete emptiness it becomes resigned to its fate. Interest in life disappears. What is left is someone who merely vegetates, without energy.

People in need of Wild Rose frequently seem half dead already, like plants that barely exist, in misery, lacking in sap. They have gone far beyond depression. They have capitulated, like people with a life sentence, and dully accepted their fate. They think their circumstances cannot be changed — their chronic illness, hopelessly stuck marriage, or unsatisfactory job. It never occurs to them that things could be different. 'It's in the family!' 'One just has to live with it.' 'It's all over as far as I'm concerned anyway.' These and similar sentences spoken in an expressionless voice, are often a puzzle to others, external circumstances not always appearing to warrant them.

People in the negative Wild Rose state are boring company and therefore tiresome, their apathetic lack of interest depressing the whole atmosphere.

The Wild Rose state has also been described as a form of 'mental anaemia', because many inhibitory mental programmes make it impossible for the person to pick up the cosmic life energies in the right quality and transform them within himself.

The Wild Rose state is not always so easily apparent, however. When it occurs at subtler levels if may even show itself in the form of frantic compensatory activity, typical examples being the 'successful manager' type.

Anyone taking Wild Rose will gradually feel his spirits revive, and begin to live again. Released, he will be able to enter into life more and more as the days go on. With vital energy increasingly flowing through him he is at last able to let all the great and little riches of life come to him, with joyful expectancy and lively interest.

Wild Rose is often a long-term Remedy, though it has also proved useful in temporary lack of energy, e.g. during psychotherapy, when the first years of life have to be integrated, also when vitality is low after burning the candle at both ends sexually, after a miscarriage, or a phase of intense work on one's own personality.

The difference between Wild Rose and Gorse with regard to hopelessness:

Wild Rose	Going along in paralyzing apathy. It never occurs to hope for anything more. Completely passive.
Gorse	Did have hopes, but is now in despair, believing his hopes finally have to be buried. Somewhat more active inwardly than Wild Rose.

The difference between Sweet Chestnut and Wild Rose as regards resignation:

Sweet Chestnut	Believes he has reached the limits of endurance, is just about to reach the limit

	where resignation sets in. Still does not give up, however.
Wild Rose	Has accepted that the limit has been passed. Has wholly or partly given up inside. More passive than Sweet Chestnut.

Wild Rose Key Symptoms
Apathy; lack of interest and ambition; resignation; has capitulated.

Symptoms Due to Energy Block
- Has resigned in one's heart, although circumstances are not that hopeless or negative.

- Feels absolutely no joy in life or inner motivation.

- Has given up making efforts to make any positive changes in one's life.

- Fatalistically resigned to everything.

- Accepts one's fate — unhappy home life, unsatisfactory job, chronic illness, etc.

- Believes one has inherited ill-health.

- Underlying hopeless sadness.

- Chronically bored, washed out, indifferent and empty.

- Does not complain of one's condition, considering it normal.

- Is always tired, with no energy at all, apathetically vegetating.

Potential Following Transformation
- Daily finds new, vital interest in life.

- Everyday life is coped with without it becoming a paralyzing routine.

- Able to follow the inner laws of life happily.

- Lives in a feeling of inner freedom and flexibility.

Supportive Measures
- Realize that it is necessary to consciously and decisively change one's negative mental programmes.

- Psychotherapy, reincarnation therapy, work with symbols.
- Physical hobbies requiring flexible reactions and improvization.

Positive Statements for Practice

'I am entitled to everything I want from life.'

'I can feel life getting more and more interesting and beautiful.'

'I am plunging into life.'

'I am developing new, positive life programmes.'

38. WILLOW,
Salix vitellina

There are many different willow species, but this one is easily recognized in winter, when its branches turn a bright orange yellow. It likes to grow on moist and low-lying ground. Male and female flowers open early in May on separate trees.

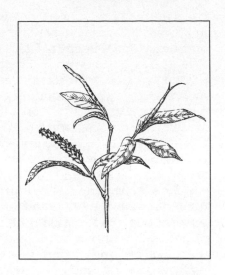

Principle

Willow relates to the soul qualities of personal responsibility and constructive thought. A person in the negative Willow state will blame everyone and everything but himself, and his thoughts tend to be negative and destructive.

On negative Willow days we rail at our fate, resenting the treatment we receive. Nor are we able to understand how others can be so cheerful and carefree; we begrudge them their good fortune and feel tempted to spoil the day for them. Each of us has such days, when we don't feel at all comfortable with ourselves. They represent a temporary negative Willow state.

Unfortunately this state may also become chronic, in which case it can have a very destructive effect on the person and his whole environment. Just as one bad apple will sooner or later cause all the others in the basket to rot, so a person in the chronic negative Willow state tends to infect others around him by being a wet blanket and spoilsport.

A person in the negative Willow state feels himself the hapless victim of a cruel fate that again and again has it in for him. 'I do not think I deserve this.' 'Life can be so unfair!' he will complain, and it never occurs to consider his own behaviour when making such accusations.

Willow is a state in which disappointments and resentment are powerfully projected onto the outside world. Essentially it is commonly seen in people who have passed the midpoint in life and unconsciously realize that only a few of their ideals and hopes have been fulfilled.

The head of department, getting on in age, now, who was passed over when a former colleague was made manager, feels that the other is looking down on him. 'Well, now that he's been advanced he can afford to ...' he'll say, his face careworn and the corners of the mouth turned down. Chronic Willow characters mutter away to themselves, having surrounded themselves with an invisible wall of negativity.

Willow types may carry a grudge for years, never putting their cards on the table and having it out. A mother-in-law, upset at heart that her daughter-in-law has moved to a home of her own with her young husband, will remain polite, but there will be underground tensions. For years, she'll never really be friendly and open towards her daughter-in-law, and when talking to her son will subtly criticize her and put her down — that is her unspoken revenge.

People who are in the negative Willow state are like a volcano that is always smouldering, ejecting clouds of acrid smoke, but never exploding.

The daughter-in-law does the shopping for her rheumatic mother-in-law and washes her curtains for her, but that is taken for granted, deserving neither mention nor praise. Willow types know well how to make demands, but are not prepared to give. This will in the long run alienate all the people who initially felt friendly and helpful towards them. They will gradually cease their efforts and withdraw.

The result is that the chronic Willow type gradually grows more isolated and embittered and on his or her part now withdraws more and more from life. Perhaps he liked to go to the bowling alley in the past, but now goes less often, because 'the new manager has been most unpleasant.' Formerly a theatre buff, he will now stay at home, 'because those new plays are either too superficial or too negative'. Whichever way you look at it, in the negative Willow state only the negative side of life will present itself. Here is a typical statement from a Willow patient who is on the road to recovery: 'I am feeling better, but not half as much as I may seem to be.' It appears as though he wanted to stop himself from letting any positive feelings arise in his heart and mind.

A person in the Willow state is a 'victim', and that provides the perfect excuse for not accepting responsibility for his own destiny. He will firmly continue to point to the outside world, absolutely refusing to acknowledge, or even consider, any connection between outside events and his own inner state.

Where does the error lie in the negative Willow state? Again it lies in a refusal on the part of the personality to accept the guidance of his soul and his Higher Self. A person in the Willow state particularly cannot agree with the outcome of such guidance, judging success in life not by inner experience but mainly according to material criteria. So she has not been able to keep her beautiful figure, he has not received the honorary doctorate, has not managed to acquire that house in the country — surely that is reason enough to rail against one's Higher Self and against fate? Unfortunately such rumbles of disapointment are not all there is to it. The personality also attempts to block all further attempts at guidance from the Higher Self by negative 'stone-walling'. Rather than work with the Higher Self it will put up passive resistance. Thus it not only harms itself but also poisons the whole environment, committing a crime against the greater whole.

Someone caught up in a persistent negative Willow state will first of all have to learn to recognize and accept his own bitterness, his own negativity. It is always necessary first to change one's attitude to one self, before anything can change on the outside. The second thing one needs to realize is that every grumbling thought adds another energy stone to the growing wall of negativity, so that one's personal sun is more and more blotted out. Everything we experience on the outside is the outcome of our own thoughts being projected outward, and every human being lives in a world he has at some stage or other thought up and created for himself. Anyone feeling himself to be a victim will inevitably sooner or later end up a victim.

Where there is much shadow there also is much light. To get out of the negative Willow state it is necessary to train oneself deliberately to concentrate on the positive side of events. Because you can always cut new shoots from the Willow tree it is not only a symbol of mourning but of infinite knowledge and a wisdom that never fails.

People in the positive Willow state come to realize that they are not the victims but the architects of their destiny, and that the human mind has unlimited facilities to work constructively for a positive future. People who have overcome their negative Willow state therefore radiate faith, calm and optimism. They know that we all have the capacity to be masters of our own fate.

It is easy to fall into a negative Willow state in the course of spiritual development, at a point when one has become aware of much that is negative but the personality is not yet strong enough to integrate this. Annoyance at oneself is then first of all projected onto the outside world, powerful prejudices develop, and there is a definite lack of co-operation.

The difference in the negative feelings of Willow and Holly:

Holly   More active and open rage, hatred, distrust etc. felt inside are given immediate expression.

Willow   More passive, with negative feelings turned inward, causing bitterness and the feeling that one is a victim. Anger smouldering beneath the surface.

Willow Key Symptoms
Unspoken resentment, bitterness, 'poor me' or 'victim of fate' attitude.

Symptoms Due to Energy Block
* Embittered attitude, resenting fate and feeling that one has been treated unjustly by life.

* Does not feel responsible for one's misfortunes, always blaming cirumstances or others.

* Thinks fate gives no recognition to what one has put into life.

* Gives up many things that one used to enjoy, resentfully withdrawing more and more from life.

* Makes demands on life, but is not prepared to give in return.

* Accepts help from others as a matter of course, in the long run alienating anyone who has tried to be helpful.

* Always stresses the negative aspect of things, often appearing a wet blanket or spoilsport.

- Morose, moody, touchy.
- At heart grudges others their better fate, good fortune or health.
- In extreme cases will even try and put a damper on the cheerful mood and optimism of others.
- Spiteful thoughts, due to bitterness felt at heart.
- Smouldering anger, unspoken, will not explode.
- Refuses in one's mind to accept one's own negativity, with the result that nothing can change.
- Does not like to admit one is feeling better when recovering from illness.

Potential Following Transformation
- Basically positive attitude, taking full responsibility for one's own fate.
- Has recognized and accepted the connection between one's thoughts and external events.
- Knows that there is a law called 'As within so without' and one therefore may attract positive or negative events; consciously makes use of this principle.
- Instead of a 'victim' becomes 'master' of one's fate.

Supportive Measures
- Consider the law of cause and effect, the concept of karma.
- Look for activities where responsibility is essential and will bring recognition and love, e.g. work with children.
- Seek the company of untroubled, cheerful people, e.g. join a choir or music group.
- Look for creative hobbies that permit self-expression and give a feeling of achievement.
- Derivative natural therapies such as fasting and lymph drainage.

Positive Statements for Practice
'I am thinking, doing and achieving positive things.'

'I can more and more see how the law of cause and effect applies to everyday life.'

'I am cleansing myself of all negative residues.'

'I am the master of my fate.'

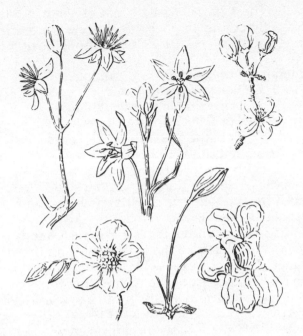

RESCUE REMEDY

'First Aid' or 'Emergency' Drops

Although not a remedy in itself, Rescue Remedy is the most widely known of the Bach Flower Remedies. It has saved countless lives in emergency situations, whilst waiting for medical help. Rescue Remedy cannot replace medical treatment. It does, however, help to prevent or quickly overcome the energetic trauma that otherwise would have serious physical consequences. In this context anything that depletes our energy is called an energetic trauma — the sudden slam of a door, bad news, or an accident involving loss of consciousness. Under those conditions, consciousness, or the subtle elements in our body, have the tendency to withdraw from the physical body and it is thus not able to initiate self-healing processes.

Rescue Remedy prevents the disintegration of the energetic system, or quickly restores it to normal. The healing process is then able to commence immediately.

It is therefore important to have Rescue Remedy in the

home medicine chest or car first-aid box, so that it may be taken immediately before an energetic trauma is expected to occur or immediately afterwards. The components of Rescue Remedy are:

Star of Bethlehem	For 'trauma' and numbness.
Rock Rose	For terror and panic.
Impatiens	For irritability and tension.
Cherry Plum	For fear of losing control.
Clematis	For the tendency to 'pass out', the sensation of being 'far away' that often precedes unconsciousness.

The stock bottle of Rescue Remedy contains all five flowers ready mixed. If Rescue Remedy is to be combined with other Flowers, it is considered as one remedy.

In case of accident or sudden illness, Rescue Remedy helps not only the 'victims' but also the bystanders and those who give assistance. The victim will unconsciously derive considerable reassurance from the feeling that those around him are calm, collected and confident. This will assist the process of recovery.

Below, some of the many occasions are listed where Rescue Remedy will prove useful in everyday life:

- When we are in mental turmoil, e.g. after a family row, on receipt of an unpleasant letter, or for children who have seen violence on television.

- For impending events such as a visit to the dentist, attending divorce proceedings, a job interview, taking one's driving test, an operation.

- If one has to work in an atmosphere of permanent stress, e.g. in a courtroom, a hospital casualty department, at an auctioneers.

Rescue Remedy should not, however, become a form of routine medication. It is indicated as first aid in greater or lesser emotional emergencies, but certainly not to make up for a lifestyle that threatens to destroy the personality through a lack of common sense.

Rescue Remedy is made up to twice the strength of all other Flower Remedies, adding 4 drops from the stock bottle to a 30ml medicine bottle.

The dosage will vary depending on circumstances.

In acute cases, four drops from the stock bottle are added to a cup of water. Sips of this are taken until the shocked feeling abates. After that, a sip is given every 15, 30 or 60 minutes.

If there is no water or other drink available, Rescue Remedy may be given undiluted, directly from the stock bottle.

If the patient is unconscious, put Rescue Remedy from the medicine bottle, or if need be also the stock bottle, on the lips, gums, temples, fontanelle, back of the neck, behind the ear or on the wrists.

If Rescue Remedy needs to be taken over a period of time, four drops are given four times daily from the medicine bottle.

Rescue Remedy may also be used externally, in compresses, packs etc., using about 6 drops from the medicine bottle to a pint of water.

For burns, sprains, stings, bumps or blows it can also be used in its concentrated form, directly from the stock bottle.

Rescue Remedy is also prepared as a cream, free from animal fat, for all external problems. It can also be helpful in massage prior to the lubricant, and it can be used as a form of precautionary application to the skin where friction is created — e.g. before running, playing tennis, etc., to help prevent soreness or blistering.

For the treatment of animals: four drops from the medicine bottle are added to the drinking water or milk or sprinkled over the food.

For large animals, 10 drops per bucket of water or, if more convenient, some drops on a cube of sugar. Often indicated remedies can be included should the need arise.

Another use for Rescue Remedy is when plants have suffered a shock — after repotting, planting out, following exposure to frost or to pests. Ten drops from the medicine bottle are added per gallon of water. The plant is watered with this as normally, at least for two or three days, or its leaves are sprayed.

The possible uses of Rescue Remedy are practically unlimited, as may be seen from the three case histories described below:

1. In wartime, a marine serving in submarines always appeared calm and relaxed, but he lost all the hair from his head and body. No medical treatment proved

effective. It was to be assumed that the loss of hair was due to suppressed fear, trauma and fright, and he was therefore given Rescue Remedy to take internally and apply as a 'hair tonic'. After a few weeks, his scalp was once again covered with short hair.

2. A young woman participating in a meditation camp cut three quarters of the way through the tip of her finger when preparing vegetables. The cut bled profusely and no doctor was immediately available. She was given a few drops of Rescue Remedy in water every few minutes, as a first-aid measure, and a pressure bandage was put on to stop the bleeding. When the bleeding had stopped, Rescue Remedy Cream was cautiously applied to the wound surfaces, and finger and fingertip were held together with a dressing. The dressing was changed every two hours. After just 15 minutes, the young woman felt no more pain, merely a slight pulsation in the finger. The dressing was changed at intervals throughout the next day. On the third day, a dressing was no longer required, for the wound had closed and was obviously healing fast. By the fifth day, the wound had healed completely. Only a fine line was left to indicate where the cut had been.

3. A little girl of 16 months pulled a tablecloth off the table. Freshly made tea caused severe burns on her head and all down the right side, and she had to be admitted to hospital. Her mother had immediately given her Rescue Remedy, also taking it herself. The result was that both were relatively calm on arrival in hospital. The doctors felt they could not offer much hope when they saw the extent of the burns. That day and throughout the following day the mother treated the burns with Rescue Remedy Cream. The doctors let her do it, for apart from pain relief there was nothing they could do at that point. By the end of the second day, the physical symptoms had largely disappeared. The skin burn areas no longer felt hot and there was no more pain. Healthy new skin showed itself on the third day — no scar tissue. The child was discharged from hospital on the fifth day — 'a miracle cure'.

Chapter 5

THE REMEDIES IN PRACTICE

A. PREPARING THE REMEDIES, BOTTLES AND DOSAGE

Preparation: The Flower Remedies are supplied in concentrated form by the Bach Centre, in stock bottles which will keep indefinitely. They need to be diluted before use, with a mixture of about three parts water to one of alcohol. Edward Bach used water from natural springs. Today still natural spring water in bottles from health food and also general stores is used. Distilled water is dead water and therefore not suitable as a vehicle.

Alcohol is only used as a preservative. It is essential, particularly at summer-time temperatures when water tends to turn bad quite quickly, and also when the drops have to be taken over a longer period of time. When a combination of Flower Remedies is to be taken just for a few days, preservation in alcohol is not absolutely necessary. Edward Bach used brandy. Cognac or similar forms of alcohol, as pure as possible, may be used instead, or cider vinegar for people who don't drink alcohol.

The standard dilution for oral medication is 2 drops from each chosen stock bottle to a 30ml (1 fl oz) medicine bottle which has been three-quarters filled with natural spring water (still) and topped up with a spoonful of brandy or cider vinegar for preservation. The mixture is then well shaken before it is used for the first time.

Brown glass bottles with drop pipette are most suitable. They are obtainable from chemists.

Dosage: Take as often as needed, but at least four drops four times daily — first thing in the morning, on an empty stomach at lunch time, on an empty stomach at about 5 p.m., and again last thing at night. The drops can be added to a baby's bottle or may be taken in a teaspoonful of water. The best method is however to put them straight on or under the tongue from the dropper. They should be held in the mouth for a moment before swallowing to gain full effect.

Care should be taken that the dropper does not come in contact with the tongue, for otherwise digestive enzymes may be transferred to the mixture in the bottle. This would affect the taste but not the efficacy of the remedies. In acute conditions much more frequent doses may be given, i.e. four drops every 10 or 30 minutes, until there are signs of improvement.

Another important alternative form of dosage, especially in acute states: Take 2 drops from each chosen stock remedy in a cup of water, fruit juice, or any beverage, and sip fairly frequently. Replenish cup to continue treatment if need be.

B. APPLICATIONS OTHER THAN BY MOUTH

Compresses. Bach prescribed compresses in addition to oral medication when there were external lesions such as skin eruptions and inflammation. 6 drops from the stock bottle are added to half a litre of water.

Baths. Many Bach therapists swear by baths containing certain Flower Remedies, e.g. Olive and Hornbeam for exhaustion. About five drops from the stock bottle are added to a full bath.

C. QUESTIONS THAT ARE OFTEN ASKED

1st Question. How long does a session with a Bach therapist normally take?

Answer. There is no rule, for everybody works in a very individual way with the Bach Flowers, some more quickly, others more slowly.

A number of practitioners using a similar approach have stated that in their experience a first session, when it is important really to get to the bottom of things, usually takes between 60 and 90 minutes. Later sessions generally take 40 to 60 minutes.

2nd Question. When is the right moment for changing to another Flower combination?

Answer. This depends on the nature of the problem, but normally not until the treatment bottle is empty, which is after 3–4 weeks. If the combination of flowers is still helpful, prepare the same combination a second time and continue using it until all symptoms have gone. (In that case the same combination is taken for 8 weeks or even longer.)

If a single new condition develops during taking this initial combination, simply add the indicated Flower Remedy to the initial combination. After that it might be necessary to reassess and either continue with the changed combination or find a new combination according to the present states of mind.

Note: There are short-term states of mind (i.e. nervousness because of taking an exam) when it is not necessary to make up a treatment bottle, because the combination is needed for a much shorter time — a week, a day or just a few hours. In such cases one can mix the drops in a glass of water and sip at intervals.

3rd Question. For how many weeks or months should treatment normally continue?

Answer. Again it is impossible to give a standard answer. It depends on the problems involved, on the age and character of the person under treatment. In acute conditions, e.g. with energetic trauma following a loss or fear of a major change, the Bach Flowers will often help within a few hours or days, particularly in younger people.

Generally speaking, one can say that if treatment is used prophylactically, before a problem takes roots, the adjustment could be quite soon, whereas the longer a condition has been allowed to develop and take hold, the more time it will take before positive changes will occur. From experience time spans of 1–20 months are possible.

People taking Bach Flower Remedies primarily for personal development and purification will go on taking them at intervals, often for years.

4th Question. How many Bach Flower Remedies may be taken at one and the same time?

Answer. According to the Bach Centre, a maximum of six or seven. The principle however is not 'the more the merrier', but rather 'less is more'.

Very much as in classical homoeopathy, the energetic impulse of a single Flower will have a deeper and more profound effect than six different impulses in a bunch. The correctly chosen single Remedy, most appropriate to the current problem, will usually also make any lesser symptoms that may be present disappear.

On the other hand experience has shown that severe emotional states may temporarily require more than one or two Remedies, even more than six.

Chapter 6

EXPERIENCES IN TREATMENT

The details given below should be considered as strictly related to the present state of experience, for times do change. This applies particularly to any figures given.

A. DIFFERENT REACTIONS

Reactions to the first dose of a Bach Flower Remedy vary as much as the individuals who take them.

In very sensitive people, the contact made between the Flower Essence and the Higher Self is apparent within a few seconds: the eyes look softer, indeed more 'soulful'. Very often a deep breath will also indicate instant relief at energy level.

People who normally cope with their experiences in dramatic fashion will also react dramatically to the Flower Remedies, e.g. with marked changes of mood, or dreams full of activity.

Some people report that they suddenly get ideas they had never had before. Others are able to make everyday decisions that just a few weeks ago they would not have thought possible. Others again notice nothing in particular to begin with, but find that after a few weeks or months they have simply become more open, stable, happy, 'more themselves'.

People who are open and interested towards the non-physical world will respond more quickly to the Flower Remedies than others who refuse to accept such ideas on principle, unconsciously wanting to silence the voice of their Higher Self over and over again, i.e. people inclined to suppress their problems.

Older people, particularly those suffering from chronic diseases, will as a rule respond less quickly to Bach Flower Remedies for they have become set in their psychic structures.

People with congenital or 'incurable' conditions always show a response as well. The new soul contact which is created will consciously or unconsciously lead to a new attitude to the illness, taking the form of greater tranquillity, peace of mind and more positive emanations. Many hospital patients in their terminal stages have been able to live through their last days in less pain, with dignity and in a feeling of greater harmony thanks to the great blessing of the Bach Flower Remedies.

B. ON THE SUBJECT OF SIDE-EFFECTS

The Bach Flowers are pure, harmonious energy frequencies that will never have side-effects. However, what may happen in some cases is a response known as 'aggravation', similar to that known in homoeopathy, when symptoms are temporarily intensified.

This means that the patient may feel worse for a short time. There is good reason for this. Imagine, a part that has been asleep or paralyzed for some time is suddenly filled with life again. A painful thought suppressed for years may suddenly come into full consciousness. Any expansion of consciousness will inevitably have its reaction in the unconscious. In naturopathy, too, a curative crisis is experienced in conjunction with toxins being cleared from the body. The same thing can happen at the level of soul and spirit when Bach Flowers are taken.

One thing is certain, however. What comes up from the unconscious will never be more than one is able to cope with at the moment. It is impossible to induce artificial curative crises with the Bach Flower Remedies, for the Flower energy merely supports the Higher Self, the Inner Physician, who always guides everything in our best interest.

C. APPARENT FAILURE

In the Bach Newsletters, J. Evans, a Bach specialist of great experience, wrote that it can happen that therapist and patient lose courage, and it seems that the Flower Remedies are getting no real response. It may even happen that patients discontinue treatment because of their disappointment and we cannot think of a reason.

When such an apparent failure occurs, we should not allow ourselves to feel too discouraged, for there are a number of factors that need to be taken into account.

Illness as a Chance to Learn

A physical illness often serves to indicate that the person needs a rest or at least has to cut down drastically on his activities. It may even be necessary to completely change one's lifestyle. Such a change would never have come into being without the illness. If the illness were made to disappear prematurely with the use of a Flower Remedy, its whole purpose would have been undone.

Wrong Moment

Another reason may be that part of the lesson to be learned from the experience of this illness has not yet been learned, and that the illness has to continue for a while yet, to offer further opportunity to learn. When treatment is later resumed at the right moment, the Flower Remedies will have the desired effect, often within a surprisingly short time.

The Patient Wants to 'Keep' His Illness

There are patients who out of inner dissatisfaction or pathological boredom keep coming back with new symptoms of minor ailments, e.g. headaches, tiredness, indefinite complaints, occasional pain etc. They insist on taking the Bach Flower Remedies, saying 'I know they'll help me.' That will indeed be the case, until the next bout of dissatisfaction appears, and 'treatment' is again required.

These people do not make rewarding patients, for they are so attached to their illness that they will unconsciously bring it back again and again.

It can indeed happen that people really do not want to get rid of their illness, for it may allow them to exercise power over others, to avoid responsibilities or arouse sympathy. They have probably already tried many different treatments, and 'none of them have really helped' — which probably will also be the case with the Flower Remedies.

The reason is that they cannot really do without their

symptoms, for they are useful to them.

Deliberate Rejection

Some people cannot in their hearts allow the Bach Flower Remedies to help them, because they simply do not wish to believe that they can help This may be the case for instance when patients have been persuaded by relatives, against their own wishes. As they are not expecting beneficial effects, and indeed in their hearts often hope there will be no effect, they deliberately set up a blockade which makes it impossible for healing forces to reach them.

Lack of Patience

Others do not allow enough time for the Bach Flower Remedies to act. Unless there are immediate and obvious results, they consider the whole treatment a failure. They fail to take into account that some illnesses, having developed over a long period of time, will also need time to clear up, step by step, and that this may indeed take considerable time. They give up too quickly, yet greater patience would have seen success.

There are many reasons and circumstances leading to illness. It is hoped that the above consideration of different aspects of the healing process will help us to realize that it is not the Bach Flowers that failed but that our understanding of so many hidden factors is still incomplete.

D. BACH FLOWERS IN CONJUNCTION WITH OTHER FORMS OF TREATMENT

As already stated, the Bach Flower Remedies will act harmoniously together with other forms of treatment, particularly all those that come under the heading of holistic medicine.

The combination of psychotherapy and Bach Therapy tends to be very fruitful as a rule. Psychotherapists describe how psychotherapy in combination with Bach therapy will be accelerated. The essential point is reached more quickly, and side issues threatening to bog things down are resolved more easily.

People not suitable for treatment often become suitable after a period of Bach Flower therapy.

Even in what are called hopeless cases, the Bach Flowers can give relief, making the patient more tranquil and amenable.

The time needed for the orthodox treatment of psychosomatic conditions can be greatly shortened if Bach therapy is given concurrently. In the treatment of chronic conditions, Bach therapy has often brought about the crucial turn in events, because the patient gained insight into the deeper-seated causes.

The Bach Flower Remedies are compatible with any other form of treatment, including high homoeopathic potencies and psychotropic drugs. The action of the former is intensified. The latter are usually gradually discontinued at the patient's own request.

E. BACH FLOWER THERAPY IN PREGNANCY, FOR BABIES AND CHILDREN

In Chapter 5 of his book *Heal Thyself* (C.W. Daniel), Edward Bach discusses the true nature of the parent-child relationship. Anyone dealing with children should take his words to heart over and over again.

Seen in its right light, parenthood is one of the greatest God-granted privileges we have. Parenthood is a matter of making it possible for a young soul to assume a physical body on this planet to achieve development. It also means giving this soul all possible spiritual, mental and physical guidance in its early years. Modern psychology now also recognizes that most mental disorders have their origin in the first seven years, and above all the first year, of life. It is perfectly evident that many problems manifesting in later life can be prevented by letting a child grow up with the Bach Flower Remedies from its very first day. That first day comes within the period of pregnancy.

Pregnancy. Bach Flower Therapy creating harmony for the expectant mother can only benefit the child, just like everything else that represents beauty and harmony during this period. There have been cases of women inclined to miscarry who reached full term for the first time after taking Bach Flower Remedies.

The method of diagnosis is no different from those used at

other times of life. Experience has shown, however, that moods change more quickly in pregnancy, and behaviour patterns one thought one had long since given up suddenly reappear with renewed intensity.

Many young women grow anxious as they get near term, developing considerable tension. In such cases, Mimulus may be considered, in extreme cases Rock Rose, and also Impatiens and Vervain. Many women who took Rescue Remedy for a few days prior to giving birth had an easy time of it, recovering quickly from the strain.

A midwife who uses the Bach Flowers with great success in Ibiza describes their effect in labour as being swift and dramatic. An example is given below:

A woman of 28, fit and of equable temperament, was doing very well until the second stage started. It continued for 90 minutes, with the young woman suddenly seeming to lose all energy and self-confidence. She was given Aspen, Mimulus, Rock Rose, Hornbeam and Oak, a few drops after every contraction. After the first dose, there was a complete change in her facial expression. She was now prepared to change position, and immediately afterwards felt that the birth was imminent.

Every birth, however straightforward, represents an energetic shock for both mother and child. Star of Bethlehem will help both of them. A mother who started taking Rescue Remedy a few days before going into labour should continue with this for a few days after giving birth. She will then of course not require Star of Bethlehem.

Infants. A question we are often asked is how to find the right Bach Flower Remedy for infants, for they are of course unable to tell us about their state of mind. It is in fact easier than one might think, for babies show their feelings quite openly.

There is the ever cheerful Agrimony baby, for instance. It will only cry when there is something seriously wrong. The Chicory baby will immediately let you know it is not pleased when its reference person ever dares to turn his or her attention to anything else. A baby made anxious and irritable by all and everything will usually respond well to Mimulus. Another type is the Clematis baby who appears to live in a world of his own. He sleeps a lot and shows little interest even in his meals.

In making the diagnosis for an infant, the Remedies taken by the parents, and particularly the mother, should also be taken into account. There are powerful energetic links at this stage of life, and some of the Flowers in the combinations used for mother and child tend to be identical.

Another interesting observation relating to diagnosis of infants is the following:

Stock bottles of all the Remedies under consideration were one after the other placed in the cradle of a sensitive infant. When the bottle contained a Flower it needed, the child would gurgle and smile, whilst reacting with whining or other signs of refusal to the others.

The dosage is normally the same for infants as for adults, overdosage being altogether impossible with Bach Remedies. Four drops from the medicine bottle are added to the infant's food four times daily. Nursing mothers take the Remedy themselves. The drops from the stock bottle have in this case of course been diluted with water only.

If the infant shows absolutely no response initially, the state of mind of the parents should serve as a guide. If the parents are fearing the worst, for instance, both parents and child are given Rock Rose. Once the doctor has been the picture will be clearer, but if there is still anxiety, Mimulus will be indicated. If the infant's condition improves so far that it again begins to show personal reactions, impatience for instance, further treatment will be based entirely on the child's emotional reactions. In the above case, Impatiens would now be indicated.

Children. Children often respond better and more rapidly to Bach Flower Remedies than adults, their behaviour patterns not being set to the same extent and mental resistance being more or less completely absent. They do not reflect much, wanting only one thing — to be well again as quickly as possible.

Children usually have no trouble at all in finding the Flower they need from among the thirty-eight stock bottles, nor do they allow others to deflect them from their choice. It is often said that children will of their own accord remind their parents when it is time to take the drops again. Like infants, children should not take too many Flowers at once. They will often also need smaller doses, and the time intervals for changing to a different Flower Remedy tend to be shorter.

There can be hardly anything more impressive and rewarding than to see how uniquely and individually children react, as long as the channel to their soul has not yet been blocked by the 'seriousness of life'. It cannot be overstressed how important it is to use Bach Flower Remedies to help children particularly at the age when they are not yet open to logical argument. They will be able to pass through the unavoidable vicissitudes and disappointments of life without suffering permanent harm in their minds and souls.

The saying 'prevention is better than cure' really applies in this case. So if young Cathy, agile and mentally always wide awake, one day comes home from school unusually tired, monosyllabic and absent-minded, and looks as though 'she's sickening for something', it is best not to leave it at that but give her some drops of Clematis and observe how she returns from her absent state to one of being all there again. There is probably no need now for her to come out in some physical illness, though if she does, experience has shown that it will be of shorter duration and less severe than in her school mates.

The Flower Remedies have been a tremendous help to many children with problems at school, as the case below illustrates:

A boy of eight was very slow at school, lagging behind in every respect. He was introverted and disinterested during lessons. His behaviour towards his class mates was unsociable, arrogant and incalculable. He would even physically attack the others and his teachers on occasion. The school finally told his parents that he could no longer be tolerated in his class and needed to be transferred to a special school. Bach therapy was the last attempt.

The therapist observed the boy for a while. He noted that he liked to play chess by himself and was always three or four moves ahead in his mind. He gave him Chestnut Bud for his poor learning performance which really was due to the mental dynamics being too powerful. Impatiens was given for the same reason, and also for his unsocial behaviour among his peers, and finally Mimulus for his generally withdrawn attitude. The boy took the combination for two

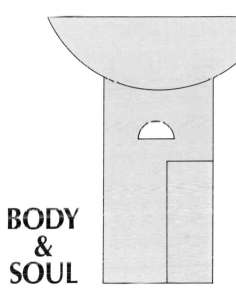

**BODY
&
SOUL**

HOLISTIC
SPIRITUAL
G R E E N
SOMATIC
GROWTH
B O O K S

52 HAMILTON PLACE
EDINBURGH EH3 5AX
Tel: 031 226 3066

weeks. His performance at school, interest in his lessons and participation improved beyond expectation. He still showed brutality towards the others, however, and now also had nightmares and walked in his sleep. Holly and Aspen were therefore added to the medication. After another two weeks he no longer showed agression towards others and was even beginning to make friends. He slept through at night without trouble.

F. BACH FLOWER THERAPY FOR ANIMALS

Animals will often react even more quickly to the Bach Flowers than humans do. Treatment is of very short duration, usually between three and ten days.

The diagnosis is made in the same way as for humans, the aim being to establish the animal's state of mind. A dog may be a Heather type, for instance, liking to hold the stage and always barking. There are Chicory dogs who constantly stick to their owner's heels, demanding attention. Cats are often Water Violet types. Mimulus will help nervous cats. Like mother and child, 'master and dog' will also often need the same Bach Flower Remedies.

Rescue Remedy has saved the lives of many animals in acute conditions such as accidents, bites, fractures, bloat and persistent vomiting.

Four drops from the stock bottle are added to the food or put directly into the mouth. Compresses made with six drops from the stock bottle to half a litre of water are helpful in the treatment of many injuries. If necessary, the drops may be applied directly from the bottle to the injured parts.

Here is an amusing case history from the archives of the Bach Centre:

A huge St Bernard was extremely sensitive to the sound of gun shots. That would not have been much of a problem had he not lived in the country, in an area where there was much hunting. Mimulus was added to his drinking water to treat his fear of noises, and gave excellent results. There was, however, a curious side-effect. Two mice lived in the house. They went out to forage at night, and in the process came in contact with the dog's drinking water. Some days later the mice suddenly appeared in broad daylight, quite unafraid, and all attempts to shoo them away failed. The dog's owner reported that she was able to get within a foot of one of the mice and yell at it loudly. In reply the mouse merely turned round and looked at her calmly, leisurely picked up a crumb of bread and trotted off. This amusing effect probably was due to the mice 'losing their inhibitions' having taken some of the Mimulus and the alcohol used to preserve the Flower Remedy.

G. BACH THERAPY FOR PLANTS

For some time, and certainly since Tompkins wrote his book *The Secret Life of Plants*, it has been known that plants, too, may suffer from shock, fear, despondency, indecision etc. Events such as repotting, drying out, or being dropped will be coped with more easily if Flower Remedies are given. As a rule Rescue Remedy should be used as the basic remedy plus any others that apply. For example, plants infested by insects will recover with Crab Apple and Agrimony, the latter for the discomfort they are unable to express. Hornbeam gives new energy to tired, sick or drooping plants.

Bach Remedy users and home gardeners have passed on the following three combinations. Ten drops from the stockbottle of each are added to a big watering can:

Growth Combination

Vine	Helps to break through the hard seed shell.
Hornbeam	Provides additional energy for the effort of growth.
Olive	Overcomes the exhaustion caused by germination and growth.

Garden Combination

Crab Apple	For pests of all kinds.
Walnut	For the transition from one growth phase to the next.
Rescue Remedy	For all environmental factors.

Cut Flowers Combination

Walnut	For the change of environment.
Wild Rose	For heads hanging down apathetically, especially in winter.
Rescue Remedy	For all environmental factors.

Chapter 7

QUESTIONS AND ANSWERS

Question: Can I achieve the same effect eating fresh gorse flowers as using the Bach Flower Remedy Gorse?

Answer: No. Eating fresh gorse flowers has an effect on the physical body, e.g. on the conduction system in the heart. The Flower Remedy Gorse is a subtle form of matter and acts at subtle levels in man, in this case on the feeling of resignation.

*

Question: Is it always essential to be consciously aware of one's own mental state if the Flowers are to have an effect?

Answer: No. The successful treatment of 'unaware' children, animals and plants shows that a neutral or positive attitude is all that is required for the treatment to take effect. It is, however, always very helpful to reflect on the principles of the Flowers which have been prescribed.

*

Question: Is it possible also to base the diagnosis on desires for the positive qualities or transformed state relating to the Bach Flowers?

Answer: No, because the Remedies can only bring back into equilibrium a state which is out of equilibrium. It is no use taking the Remedies as long as one is in harmony.

For example: a person who is not jealous or suspicious could not take Holly to prevent himself from ever feeling jealous or suspicious. The Remedies are meant to cater for those who suffer from an 'overdose' of an emotion, not as a preventative. A non-worrier cannot take White Chestnut to prevent himself from ever having worries. He could need it, however, when he finds that his mind becomes tormented by worries, preferably at the first sign of this.

*

Question: What is the difference between type-remedies and helping remedies?

Answer: Type-remedies, or basic remedies correspond to potentials which are to be found in their personality's character structure. They might be needed again at intervals in the course of one's life. Helping remedies assist the personality to reharmonize acute negative states of mind that are not characteristic but temporary (e.g. impatience before a trip, or apprehension before a court-case).

Each of the 38 Bach Flower Remedies can act as a type-remedy or a helping-remedy.

*

Question: Does there always have to be a first or primary reaction with Bach therapy?

Answer: No. Aggravations or intensified symptoms are very uncommon and depend on the character of the person and the situation in which he finds himself. In general it can be said that aggravations are always a good sign, for they will once more put a spotlight on the problems involved, thus increasing the motivation for change.

For example, a woman who had separated from her husband years ago but had never been able to accept the separation properly and digest it, temporarily found it all coming up again when she had taken her first dose. She saw once more, very clearly, that she never wanted to go through anything like her former marriage again. Having made this decision, she began to develop behaviour patterns which prevented her from getting herself into the same kind of situation again.

Another example is a publisher who got a bad attack of 'flu when he had taken his first dose of Bach Flowers, and had to stay in bed for ten days. But that was exactly what he had not allowed himself to do for ten years, feeling that he could not leave his business in the lurch.

Dr Alec Forbes observed that patients who had made a very sudden change from psychotropic drugs to Bach Flowers would sometimes complain of reactions such as dizziness, headache and mood swings. In his experience these are not first reactions to the Bach Flowers, but withdrawal symptoms following the discontinuation of the other drugs.

*

Question: What can be done when a very strong aggravation develops?

Answer: Rescue Remedy, taken in addition for some days will deal with this.

In really extreme cases, which are most uncommon, it is advisable to discontinue the Bach Flower Remedies for a day or two, and then start again, reducing the dose if necessary. It is, however, much better to go through with the first reaction, for it is an awareness crisis. Until now, any such crisis has always passed quickly.

*

Question: What might be the reason for the sudden feeling that one does not want to take even a single drop more, when before one has been taking a combination of Bach Flower Remedies with regular enthusiasm?

Answer: This is usually a sign that at this point the Flowers have reached their maximum effect. The cycle has come to an end. Some people will also suddenly 'lose' their medicine bottle or simply forget to take the drops.

*

Question: What may be done when treatment comes to a dead stop after some time, and one has the feeling of making no further progress?

Answer: Edward Bach recommended Holly and Wild Oat to 'open things up'. Holly for the more extrovert energetic type, Wild Oat for people who are more passive. Star of Bethlehem has also proved effective as a general catalyst and 'personality integrator'. When the person treated loses his initial enthusiasm and suddenly feels discouraged and doubtful, Gentian will restore the conviction that such problems can be overcome.

*

Question: How does it happen that someone who has been taking the Bach Remedies happily and with success for some months will break off treatment with absolute suddenness?

Answer: The treatment has probably brought him very close to one of his most essential problems, and he would now be called upon to make a very major change, e.g. give up a partnership. He may be unable or unwilling to make such a change at this point.

*

Question: Do the Bach Flower Remedies act in the same way in all continents and all climates?

Answer: Experience shows that the Bach Flower Remedies are used with the same success in India, Australia or South America as in Europe. The archetypal human soul concepts such as love and hate or guilt and regret addressed by the Flower Remedies are on a collective level of consciousness, common to all people and races.

*

Question: Two different Bach therapists 'prescribed' two different combinations of Bach Flower Remedies for me on one and the same day. Some of the Flowers in both combinations are the same, others quite different. Was one of the combinations wrong?

Answer: Assuming both therapists are equally well qualified, we may assume that both diagnoses were correct.

The process of diagnosis always involves communication at an energetic level between two individuals which is never identical. Every person making a diagnosis will naturally perceive certain problems in the character of the other person with particular clarity, these being those he has himself lived through and integrated. These then are the problems he can concentrate on and where he is most able to help and prescribe the flowers needed.

Since most of us have more than one problem at the same time, both diagnoses may be correct.

Another reason may be that one therapist perceives more the processes that are in the forefront, whilst the other is considering more those below the conscious threshold. In theory, the two therapists could arrive at completely different diagnoses in such a case.

A patient should always only consult a single therapist at a time. Otherwise considerable unrest will result in the energetic system and no real development can take place.

*

Question: Two ladies I know were both suffering from chronic irritative cough, and years of medical treatment had given no relief. One was prescribed Star of Bethlehem and Chestnut Bud, the other Beech, Mimulus and Heather. Does this mean all five Flowers are good for chronic irritative cough?

Answer: No. The Flower Remedies are generally not used directly for physical complaints but for the negative states of mind or moods which might hinder the recovery from a physical complaint. In this light each of the 38 Flower Remedies could have an 'indirect' influence on the specific negative states of mind depending on the psychological history of the individual personality.

In the first case, the cough had been triggered by a shock experienced when she was younger (Star of Bethlehem). She had however failed to draw any conclusions from this (Chestnut Bud). The result was that she would unconsciously be getting herself over and over again into similar shock situations and then have to 'cough them away'.

The second patient was a very sensitive person (Mimulus), but also highly critical of others (Beech), and on top of this rather ego-centered (Heather). What she had experienced through the day in contact with other people — and she was always relating it all too much to her own person — had to be 'coughed up' again at night.

*

Question: I have become more sensitive since taking the Bach Flowers, particularly in my reactions to atmospheric variations and changes in the weather. What causes this?

Answer: The Bach Flower Remedies encourage the development of greater awareness. Things you previously did not take much note of are registered more consciously now, reacting according to your character. Another factor is that one is also less stable in the physical sense when going through a phase of increased psychic activity, with many mental structures undergoing changes. These phases are most valuable, for it is exactly in such states that changes can really take place. Recognizing and accepting such unstable states as positive transition stages, you will automatically find the right ways and means to cope with them.

A Bach Flower many people find helpful in coping with changes in the weather is Scleranthus.

*

Question: I have a friend who is using the Bach Flower Remedies to treat all kinds of minor, passing upsets and ailments, e.g. when she's got out of bed the wrong way or happens to feel guilty at having yelled at her daughter. Is this reasonable, or does it reduce the effectiveness of the Remedies when they are really needed?

Answer: Yes, it is quite in order to treat everyday ups and downs and mood changes as soon as they arise. Whether one wants to do this depends on the inner attitude and degree of awareness. Bach used to say: 'If cold, put on a cardigan and, if hungry, have something to eat; if you wake up one day lacking in confidence take some drops of Larch.'

*

Question: We hear so much about cancer these days and other fatal illnesses. I am desperately afraid that I might also get them. Is there a Bach Flower Remedy against this fear?

Answer: Yes, indeed several. Fear is one of the main causes of illness altogether. Fear persisting for a long time will increasingly isolate us from our souls and therefore from the stream of divine energy that lends us natural resistance to disease. Generally speaking it may be said that Mimulus has often proved helpful in the treatment of cancerophobia, but it is better not to consider this fear in such an isolated fashion, and rather find the combination that expresses your character, continuing treatment for some time.

*

Question: I have been taking Bach Flower Remedies for some weeks, for inner sadness and tension which I have had for some time. My moods have improved, but I have suddenly developed eczema and a discharge. I want to stop the drops now, because they obviously are not good for me. Is that correct?

Answer: No. You are mistaken in transferring the experiences and reservations you have collected through years of ordinary drug treatment onto the Flower Remedies.

The Flower Remedies act quite differently from the usual medicaments. They provide for spiritual, mental and also physical cleansing and development. The change in mood, the skin eruption and discharge indicate that the cleansing process has been set in motion at all levels. If you persevere now, the physical signs of cleansing will soon pass. You should also remember, however, that conditions that have taken years to develop cannot be undone from one day to the next. Give yourself time, and follow your own cleansing process with interest and love. This will accelerate it.

*

Question: I suffer from a stomach complaint that runs in the family. The doctors say I have to live with it. Is there any point in a Bach Flower Therapy in my case?

Answer: Most certainly. But rather than using such therapy to counter the condition, you will now be able, to come to terms with the illness at another level with the aid of the Bach Remedies. You will find out what your sick stomach wants to tell you, and discover the character weaknesses in yourself and your family that relate to this. Even character traits that are 'in the family' need not be taken for granted and accepted. On the contrary, they are a challenge to develop your own personality. Having realized this, your attitude to your illness will change, you will find it easier to live with it and there will very likely also be quite considerable improvement.

*

Question (from a member of an alternative religious group): Our Guru says the goal is to give up our own ego, to merge into cosmic energy. What point is there in that case in working with the Bach Flowers to develop one's character? Would it not be better simply to ignore our faults and do as the Guru says?

Answer: That is a very common misconception today. You can only give up what you actually have, and not what you have never developed. Anything ignored, with no conscious energy directed towards it, cannot develop, but merely harden. Most religions are in agreement that in the first place, it is our self-chosen task on this planet to develop the personality by expanding awareness and recognizing the divine laws, making it into a superb instrument that will permit each of us to make our own, unique contribution to the progress of the greater whole. The experience gained in the process, coupled with a fundamentally positive attitude, will of its own accord refine the personality more and more. As a result, the personality will develop what Edward Bach referred to as Virtues.

The personality may consider the suggestions made by masters relating to development, but it has to follow its own inherent laws. Genuine contact with God is possible only by uniting one's own refined personality with the soul. That is the only way in which we can 'merge into the cosmos'.

*

Question: Homoeopaths are constantly discovering new remedies that were not known in Hahnemann's day. Is the Bach system also capable of extension?

Answer: No. Shortly before he died, Edward Bach said that his system of 38 Flowers covered all essential soul qualities in man and that it was complete in itself. The system therefore needs neither extension nor completion.

*

Question: Could successful Bach Flower Therapy only be a placebo effect?

Answer: No. The Bach Flowers have been shown to produce reliable results in 'unaware' animals and young children. This should convince even sceptics that this is not a matter of imagined results, but of a direct effect, though at a very subtle level.

*

Question: Do the energy vibrations of one stock bottle affect those of another when two open bottles are placed side by side?

Answer: No. It makes no difference if bottles are put side by side open or closed.

*

Question: I accidentally touched the pipette of the stock bottle with my tongue. Will this spoil the contents of the bottle?

Answer: No. The Flower Extracts will not be affected by this.

*

Question: Some people say it is possible to top up the stock bottles again and again with brandy, and that this will not weaken their effect, so that one can go on with them for ever. Is that correct?

Answer: No. There must be some misunderstanding here. The Flower Remedies will keep for an unlimited period under normal storage conditions, but of course only in the original formulation.

*

Question: I accidentally added one drop more from the stock bottle than necessary when making up a mixture for use. Does this mean the mixture in the medicine bottle is too strong, or can it be used?

Answer: You will be able to use it. The water in the medicine bottle is merely the vehicle for the Flower energy, and overdosage is quite impossible with the Bach Remedies. The exact size or number of the drops therefore has not so much relevance with regard to their action. This is also evident from the fact that made-up remedy mixtures (2 drops of each remedy to a 1 ounce or 30ml bottle) are just as effective as taking 2 drops of each chosen remedy in a glass of water as a daily dose.

*

Question: I have heard that Bach Flower Remedies may also be prescribed according to one's astrological chart. Is this true?

Answer: The general answer to this rather general question has to be No. Every case and everything that happens at any moment is unique, and the best possible diagnosis will be achieved only at the moment when the person seeking treatment and the therapist are face to face. Anything else may do more harm than good.

*

Question: I find it difficult to accept the moral judgements that easily tend to come up in connection with a Bach diagnosis. Would it not be possible to handle this in a more neutral way?

Answer: There are two aspects to this. Of course no one has the right to judge and put a value on the behaviour of others, for we never know what laws another soul is following. As Bach himself once put it, most impressively, anything bad is merely something that in itself is good but is in the wrong place or at the wrong time. This does not mean, however, that we should close our eyes to evidently destructive character traits in others. That in itself would also constitute destructive behaviour, paradoxical as this may seem. If we consider life on this planet to be one great process of learning from each other and maturing, everyone of us is challenged not to refuse the learning processes that come towards him, but to accept them, not only for oneself, but also for the sake of our fellow human being and of the greater whole. It means that we must seriously respond to evidently destructive behaviour in another person, to the best of our ability, so that we do not deprive them of the opportunity to learn which they are unconsciously looking for.

*

Question: Do the Bach Flower Remedies have a more intensive effect if given by injection?

Answer: No. The Remedies work at more subtle levels of human energy, and injection into the physical body would offer no advantage. On the contrary. Injection is a comparatively 'invasive' method of application, and as such totally alien to the subtle way these Remedies work. Injection should definitely not be used.

*

Question: Is it possible to prepare the Flower Remedies without any alcohol for the treatment of alcoholics?

Answer: The original mother tinctures of the Bach Flower Remedies have to contain alcohol. But, however, the following method may be used to make the drops the patient is taking practically alcohol-free:

In making up the treatment, bottle cider vinegar is used instead of alcohol. When two drops from a stock bottle are added to a 30ml medicine bottle containing water and cider vinegar, the alcohol content will be approximately 0.16%. The four-drop dose from the medicine bottle is not put directly on the tongue, but added to a glass of mineral water or fruit juice from the refrigerator. The alcohol content is now so low that it can no longer be measured.

*

Question: In what form are the Remedies available?

Answer: Stock bottles are available in complete sets of all 38 Remedies plus Rescue Remedy, or individually. They come in two sizes:

    10ml = approx. 140 drops (sufficient for about 60 medicine bottles)

    30ml = approx. 320 drops (sufficient for about 180 medicine bottles)

Under normal storage conditions the contents of the stock bottles will keep indefinitely. Rescue Remedy is also available as Rescue Remedy Cream (27g tubes).

FURTHER READING

The Twelve Healers, Edward Bach, 1933.

Heal Thyself: An Explanation of the Real Cause and Cure of Disease, Edward Bach, 1931.

The Medical Discoveries of Edward Bach, Nora Weeks, 1940.

The Illustrated Handbook of the Bach Flower Remedies, Philip M. Chancellor, 1971.

Introduction to the Benefits of the Bach Flower Remedies, Jane Evans, 1974.

The Bach Remedies Repertory, F.J. Wheeler, 1952.

Dictionary of the Bach Flower Remedies, T.W. Hyne Jones, 1975.

A Guide to the Bach Flower Remedies, Julian Barnard, 1979.

All the above books are published by C.W. Daniel Co. Ltd., Saffron Walden, Essex, England. As well as through bookshops they are obtainable from The Bach Centre (see Useful Addresses).

Flowers to the Rescue, Gregory Vlamis, Thorsons, 1986.

USEFUL ADDRESSES

For those who wish to pursue the subject further, the Bach Centre can provide general information and order forms relating to the individual or complete sets of stock remedy concentrates and all published books and other material on the subject. Please include an sae with your enquiry.

The Bach Flower Remedies Ltd
The Bach Centre
Mount Vernon
Sotwell
Wallingford
Oxon   OX10 0PZ
England
(Tel. 0491 39489/34678)

Official distributors of the Bach Centre are:

United States of America/Canada

Ellon (Bach USA) Inc.
PO Box 320
Woodmere
NY 11598
(Tel. 516-825-2229)

Australia

Martin & Pleasance Wholesale Pty Ltd
PO Box 4
Collingwood
Victoria 3066
(Tel. 419-9733)

Nonesuch Botanicals Pty Ltd
PO Box 68
Mt Evelyn
Victoria 3796
(Tel. 762 8577)

Holland

Holland Pharma
Postbus 37
7240 AA Lochem
(Tel. 05730-2884)

Denmark

Camette
Murervej 16
6700 Esbjerg
(Tel. 05-155444)

Germany, Austria, Switzerland

Mechthild Scheffer HP
Bach Centre – German Office
Eppendorfer Landstrasse 32
2000 Hamburg 20
(Tel. 040/46 10 41)

INDEX